Parenting Happy Healthy Children

KAREN OLNESS, M.D.
Mother & Pediatrician

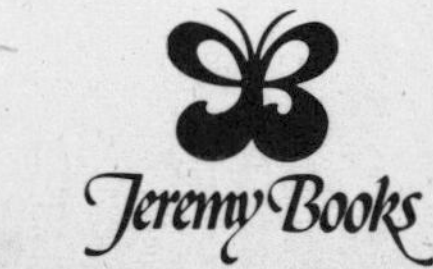

5624 Lincoln Drive, Minneapolis, Minnesota 55436

PARENTING HAPPY HEALTHY CHILDREN

A Jeremy Book / Published by arrangement with Karen Olness, Eden Prairie, Minnesota.

Originally published under the title RAISING HAPPY HEALTHY CHILDREN.

ISBN 0-89877-032-7

Printed in the United States of America

ABOUT THE AUTHOR

Dr. Karen Olness is Director of Medical Education and Research at the Minneapolis Children's Health Center and Associate Professor of Pediatrics at the University of Minnesota Medical School. She is a fellow of the American Academy of Pediatrics and past president of the Northwestern Pediatric Society. During the period described in the book, Karen Olness raised three young children full-time, and practiced medicine part-time in Laos, Kenya and Washington, D.C., where her husband served in the U.S. Foreign Service. Her work ranged from missionary medicine and international public health to a suburban private practice and a position on the medical faculty at George Washington University. Shortly after the years described in the book, she and her husband traded roles—he assumed primary child-care responsibility while she became more active in teaching and practicing pediatrics. They also adopted a fourth child, who almost entirely escaped the dubious distinction of being recorded in this book.

To my parents
whose faith in happy
outcomes for their five children
was never dimmed by a
lack of worldly goods.

Acknowledgments

The children deserve special acknowledgment, not only because it was their existence that made this book possible, but also because they cheerfully gave their permission to us to publish stories of their childhood. I am aware that there may be an interval during their adolescence when they will wish this had not happened. For that I beg their forgiveness and trust that in the end they will be glad to show the book to our grandchildren.

I thank my husband for being so much involved in the rearing of the children, for his encouragement in this project from the time the diary writing began, and for the many hours he has given to editing the manuscript for publication. I am grateful to numerous friends, relatives and colleagues who have read drafts of the manuscript over the years and contributed their suggestions and criticisms.

Karen Olness, M.D.

CONTENTS

Foreword by Donald W. Delaney, M.D.

The way we raise our children today may have a greater effect on the future of our own society than the total advances of technology, medicine, transportation and communication. However, we place comparatively little importance on training parents in child rearing, on research into more ideal methods to fulfill this responsibility, and on support of the family unit, which suffers from much criticism.

Time was when children were incorporated into the family immediately after birth with the expectation that as soon as possible they would carry their fair share of the work. Chores were assigned in a progressive fashion in keeping with the developmental skills of each child. The completion of these tasks not only benefited the other members of the family, but also gave the child a feeling of being an integral part of the family, a sense of contributing to others, a feeling of accomplishment and a spirit of independence.

The family no longer depends upon the child to contribute a fair share of the load. Automatic dishwashers, clothes washers and dryers, pre-packaged food and piped-in fuel have replaced tasks previously carried out in some way by the children within a family. Today the accomplishment of lessons —swimming, dancing, riding, music, tennis—and leagues—baseball, football, soccer—are the expectations of parents for their children. Frequently the child becomes further dependent upon his parents as chauffeurs to carry out these expectations, while he or she spends much less time fulfilling tasks from which the family derives immediate benefit. The child may develop a view of self as a recipient of all family efforts, a state which appears to foster dependence and lower self-esteem.

Time was when the family unit consisted of grandparents, uncles, aunts and intimate lifelong friends who helped in the tasks of child rearing, reinforcing the parental goals, sharing in the provision of love, comfort and recognition of young parents and children alike. Babysitting was provided not only free, but by a known, loved, respected and obeyed adult relative. Time was, also, when each child was known as an individual within his immediate community, called by his or her given name, encouraged, and nudged back into line if a transgression occurred without the threat of calling the police.

The family of today does not have this extended family and neighborhood support. Job demands, desire for promotion bringing increased prestige and salary, and the anticipation of a new neighborhood as exciting and more promising have led to frequent moves of families. The development of intimacy between neighbors is avoided because of the inevitable painful separation. The father frequently is not involved in his community because his work is outside that neighborhood, and the pressures of work and commuting continuously leave him with little energy and time to develop a sense of community. Parents of today's children feel this loss of support and this isolation which can be so devastating. Parents recognize the inequity in society's demands for many years of preparation and continuous inservice education for their job or career, and none for that important job of raising their children. Child-rearing techniques have been left to chance, dependent upon the feelings of the moment, the way the parents were raised as children, and the norms of the immediate community and culture wherein the family resides. These same parents are alarmed by the acts of violence, the drug and alcohol addiction, shoplifting, dropouts and runaways which they witness and hear about among our youth. Insecure in their own child-rearing practices which they learned from their parents, and recognizing that these methods were learned during different times, with different societal norms, and frequently in different cultures—parents are reaching out for help and searching for support. Many articles and books have been written offering good advice; but while attempting to carry out this advice, parents have been distracted from showing their affection by that special relaxed smile, the look of encouragement, the spontaneous hug and kiss—or, on the other hand, their disapproval by that frown or warning tone of voice.

Dr. Karen Olness has shared with us her experiences as a mother and has utilized her expert pediatric and insightful knowledge in relating the growth and development of her children. She and her husband are truly remarkable parents who have combined familial, cultural and scientific factors in arriving at their own child-rearing techniques. I can attest to the fact that they have been very successful with their four exciting, intelligent, lovable children—each a different and personable individual. What genetic factors are involved can only be distinguished by the physical characteristics of these children. One can ask if they picked their third child from that orphanage in Laos because she was the prettiest, the most alert, and so on. I think not, because I had the occasion to examine her shortly after she became a member of the family. How she and their fourth child, the other adopted non-white member of this four-child family, have developed is an exciting revelation, although I recognize that it is not the purpose for which the book was written.

Foreword

Dr. Olness has written an exciting book, brought alive by the incorporation of her own family; a human book in which she confesses to her lack of training as a mother and reflects on her mistakes; a helpful book which not only gives sound advice to concerned parents but, above all, also gives parents the much needed permission to relax and be themselves. Affection and approval of children correct the mistakes of inconsistency.

Donald W. Delaney, M.D.

Associate Director,
Patient Care and Educational Coordination
Children's Hospital National Medical Center

Professor,
Child Health and Development
The George Washington University
School of Medicine

Washington, D. C.

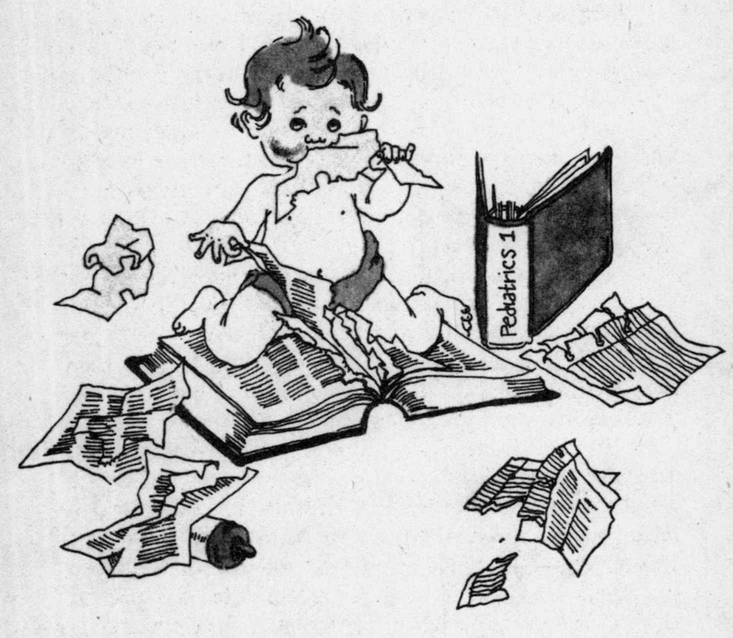

I have found that my own experiences as a mother have helped me more in counseling parents than any of the theoretical child rearing methods I had studied.

INTRODUCTION

Before I was a mother I was a pediatrician. I knew a lot about sick children and a little about well children.

When our first baby was born eleven years ago, I was preparing for the pediatric board exams. I remember breast feeding Peter while balancing on the arm rest a ponderous *Textbook of Pediatrics* which weighed as much as my baby. My mind was crammed with information on endocrine disturbances and immuno-deficiences and hundreds of other subjects a pediatrician must understand to be certified. Feedback from my patients and peers gave me assurance that I was a good pediatrician.

But the child at my breast was something different. The "objective" data of my profession did not cover the rearing he would need. Even though patients were already asking me for advice on child rearing, I was aware that this was not a subject I understood well. Nor did many of the other new pediatricians who were my peers.

With time I learned, as do most pediatricians, that it is easier to understand and solve the intricate problems of children's diseases than it is to understand and solve the daily dilemmas of child rearing. I realized also that the subject which probably should dominate the dialogue between parents and pediatricians in the United States is the rearing of our children rather than the curing of their physical ills. Physical ills are important and require attention. For most children, fortunately, they only occur occasionally. Management decisions regarding child rearing must be made daily. The quality of these decisions can affect not only the general development of the child, it can also impinge on the incidence and course of certain physical ills such as accidents, nutritional deficiencies, bedwetting, etc.

My experience taught me that the neat theories of child rearing could easily fall apart in specific situations depending on the particular child, the particular parent, and a host of other variables. Neither parents nor their children are consistent. If we forget this, the "methods" can leave us confused, anxious and guilt-ridden. I have recommended books on parenting to parents in the past, only to have some of them return with the book in one hand and a troubled child in the other to say it didn't work:

"I know the cause of all his problems is that he's a middle child, and I'm an oldest child. I feel so guilty. I try, but I'm not making it." Or,

"I put the pennies in the purse every morning, and I took them out whenever she had a tantrum. On the third morning she grabbed the purse and threw all the pennies into the toilet. How come Behavior Mod doesn't work for us?" Or,

"I've tried the 24-hour toilet training routine four times, and he still isn't trained. What do I do now?"

Proponents of any method can find a perfectly logical reason why the method didn't work in a particular situation: You didn't persist long enough or you misinterpreted the book or you implemented the method incorrectly. If the method is one that has seemed to work in our own particular situation, it is very difficult not to project the same method on others. This is neither realistic nor sympathetic. No method is gospel. Any method can work wonders at times and flop at other times.

So I have become less dogmatic and, I hope, more sympathetic in my talks with parents. I have found that my own experiences as a mother have helped me more in counseling parents than any of the theoretical child-rearing methods I had studied.

My own experience, and that of the many parents with whom I have talked over the years, has convinced me that there is rarely a single solution to a child-rearing problem. Most families have innate abilities to develop their own solutions to situations they perceive as problems. Neither the perception of the problem nor its solution may necessarily make much sense to the rest of us.

It is useful, however, to share our experiences, because there are attitudes which we can learn from one another that make it easier to create our own solutions. We can see what happens when someone gets uptight about a situation and compare that with the outcome when someone else stayed relaxed and used common sense in a similar situation. We can discover that many of the situations we perceive as problems are, on closer examination, found to hinge on questions of definition and tolerance. If this is the case, then the solution might involve primarily a change in our definition of a "problem" or an adjustment of our level of tolerance.

For example, if parents become accustomed to the ravenous appetite of their baby prior to age one, they may regard it as a problem when the baby "doesn't eat a thing anymore" sometime during the second year. If, on the other hand, they know there is a natural reduction in the appetite after age one, they need not regard the feeding change as a problem.

Or if one or both parents grew up as only children in neat homes, they may find it difficult to tolerate the geometric progression of messiness which occurs with each additional child in a family. They must adjust their level of tolerance for messiness if they are to enjoy family life.

The sharing of our experiences allows us to discover that others can be just as overwhelmed by the demands of parenting as we. There's comfort in that simple realization. The sharing of our experiences allows us to discover that others have the same yearning for quick, certain solutions that we have, and that it takes time for most of us to learn how very few are the certainties in parenting.

Like many mothers I had kept an elaborate record of the development of my first baby, Peter. I loved to bore my friends and relatives with details of his progress. The records of my second baby, Anne, were kept more haphazardly; and the baby book for Joy, our third child, might have been slim indeed had I not become seized with the idea of keeping a diary on all three of them. I thought a diary might shed some light on the child development theories and child-rearing techniques which I had been recommending to parents of my patients.

I persisted with the diary on an almost daily basis for five years (the diary continues to the present, albeit with less frequent entries), collecting handwritten notes, typed entries, and, more frequently, cassette tapes of dictation. During midnight leisure periods, I would transcribe a week or two of dictated tapes.

This book is based on excerpts from that diary, with commentary from the perspective of four years after the diary ended. The diary excerpts are unedited. I confess that I would have liked to ignore or change or repress some of them. In fact, my husband and I realized that we had forgotten many of the incidents recorded in the diary. We now find it easier to understand how grandparents can insist that "You were completely toilet trained by eight months," or "None of my children ever did anything like that," or "I never spanked any of my children."

I selected the diary excerpts based on an analysis of the subjects that came up most frequently in the diary and a study of the most frequent questions that parents had raised with me during well-baby and pre-school check-ups. Some entries fit no category whatever and were included just for fun.

A diary format offers a useful way to look at child development. It gets away from the theoretical models and allows us to encounter questions as they come up in the helter-skelter of a household with small children.

A diary does impose one important element of structure which is the element of sequential development. This means that the natural sequence of development which occurs for each child becomes apparent as the diary progresses. Babies babble before they talk, they have tantrums in the process of learning about independence, and they must touch and taste their world before they can read books about it. If portions of this natural sequence are omitted, the results might be harmful to later development.

We have tried to eliminate from the book the personal biographical information that usually adorns a diary. The questions and problems we were recording were not related just to our own specific circumstances. We believe they could be widely shared in our Western culture.

Briefly, however, during the diary years I was practicing medicine—part-time mostly—and I was the primary caretaker of our children. My husband was in the U.S. Foreign Service. Most of the record occurs while we were living in Washington, D.C., but the diary begins while we were serving in Vientiane, Laos, followed by a year-and-a-half in Nairobi, Kenya. My work ranged from missionary medicine to international public health, to a suburban private practice, to academic medicine. Shortly after the end of the five years of the diary, my husband and I traded roles. He assumed primary responsibility for the children as I became more active in teaching pediatrics. And we adopted a fourth child, who almost entirely escaped the dubious distinction of being recorded in this book.

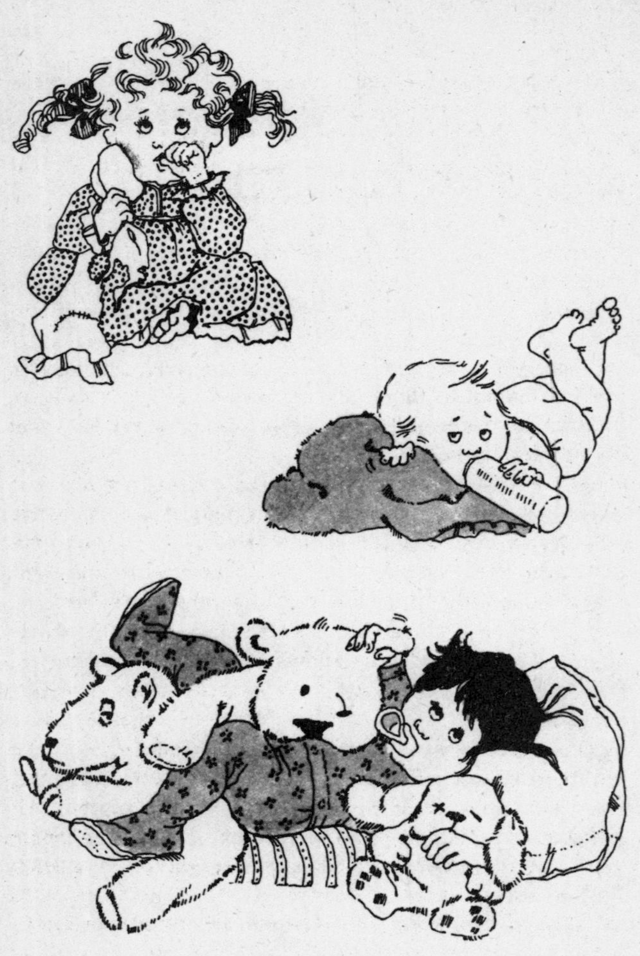

There is no simple answer to the question of pacifiers. Sucking urges vary from infant to infant.

1
Life with children aged infant to three

During the first year of this diary our children ranged in age from infant to three, and we learned to live with three children in diapers. It was a heady experience for older parents like ourselves.

In the diary our children are called Peter, Anne and Joy. This record starts when Peter was two-and-a-half, Anne had just turned one, and our adopted daughter, Joy, had just joined the family at age six months. She was malnourished, weak and ill with chronic diarrhea and an ear infection.

Normal Chaos

The mixture of confusion, happiness, anger, joy, insecurity, fulfillment and fatigue of a household with small children will be understood by parents who are living with it. I do not think any "expert" who has not personally experienced it will ever understand it adequately. Here is how a day started:

> July 19—Joy woke us at 6 a.m. Peter and Anne were up by 6:30. At 6:45 Daddy found Peter sitting on our bedroom carpet with pants full of stool and a trail of the same leading from the playroom. I heard Daddy scolding and tried to doze on and ignore the whole

> scene. I finally got up, gave Peter a spank and cleaned up the whole mess. Breakfast was at 7:15. Anne finished an enormous helping and begged for more. Peter ate happily in the high chair while Joy was in the playpen enjoying her first bottle of the day. Peter got down and started pulling books from the shelf. Anne imitated. By 8:00 we had all the books back on the shelf and were starting to dress Peter. It was his nursery school day. He resisted dressing, as he sometimes does. I asked, "Don't you want to go to school?" He said, "No." Anne was in the tub drinking bathwater. Joy had her first bowel movement of the day.

Parents of small children know that the start of this particular day was not unusually chaotic. But to an outsider or even a father who is not involved, it may seem quite overwhelming. Common advice from those who do not understand the process goes like this: "If you'd only get organized, the household would run smoothly and you wouldn't be so tired." There were times when I believed that advice and felt guilty. But it was not useful advice. What worked best for us was to reduce, if possible, the number and kinds of things that we would regard as problems. This mental exercise made it easier to cope.

On this particular day the diary shows that the pace continued without interruption for a little over fourteen hours. Here is the end of the day:

> By 6:45 p.m. Anne was crabby and sleepy. She took her one bottle for the day and consumed it in sixty seconds. This was followed by fearsome yelling. I tried to ignore her and then to distract her with storybooks. Then Joy joined the screeching. When I held her, Peter

> became jealous and tried to destroy the infant chair. Daddy got home from work, and we had parents' supper. Anne ate again, sitting on Daddy's lap. Peter also ate a second supper. At 7:50 we all went upstairs. Anne was rocked to sleep. Peter fell asleep with Daddy lying beside him, and Joy went to sleep with her bottle. 8:15 p.m. Bliss!

It is the genius of the human animal and other species that we most of us can adapt to the extraordinary demands of raising children when the task confronts us. Rereading our diary and talking with new parents, I am amazed at how routinely we can adapt to a steady pace of days like the one described here and come away from them with happy memories.

Do we try to do too much? I think all the time we can spend with the children in those first years is very well spent. But I suspect we do too many other things. While the children are napping we frantically scrub and bake and polish. We keep our houses cleaner than our mothers and grandmothers ever did, and we have less help from extended families than they had. Things went better for our family when we were able to spend some of those nap times restoring our own souls as the kids were restoring theirs.

Constant Watch

A luxury we discovered a few years later was the realization that, as the kids got older, we no longer needed to be on constant alert for them. But for several years the routine described in the diary was one of constant watch. Here's how it went in the middle of the same day:

July 19—Back home, the girls had naps—Anne for 30 minutes and Joy for an hour. I played with them until 11:00 and we went to get Peter. He insisted on sitting in my lap and helping to steer the car.* Lunch was at 11:30. Peter spilled his milk, wet his pants, then adamantly refused the idea of a nap. Finally he fell asleep at 12:45. I then discovered to my horror that Anne had climbed halfway up the stone staircase by herself. Joy napped well; but Anne stayed awake and active, moving objects from their rightful places and pushing an old walker up and down the playroom. Joy awakened happy and was trying earnestly to sit alone and put weight on her legs. I cleansed her draining ear. After snacks I put on the Swan Lake record. Peter and Anne danced. But when my back was turned they pulled out the books again. Supper at five; then baths for each of the children. While I was hunting for towels, Peter found the shampoo and squirted it in the eyes of Anne and Joy. What grief! After washing their eyes, I gave Joy a pacifier. Anne kept after it, so I gave one to each of the others. Peter, who had never used the gadget, lay down contentedly to imitate Joy. Anne was dissatisfied until she had exchanged her pacifier with Joy's.

There are many things we do to childproof our homes—putting a gate on a hazardous stairway or setting our valuable objects well out of reach. Children still need watching. And watching them for twelve to fourteen hours day after day becomes tedious even for child researchers. Anyone who doubts this should try it for a month.

It helps if you can share the chore.

*It may help the shocked reader to know that the maximum speed possible on that particular road was ten miles per hour. The author does not approve of children sitting on laps in cars—but she has also been inconsistent in the face of childish pleasure.

Pacifiers and Thumb-sucking

There is no simple answer to the question of pacifiers. Sucking urges vary from infant to infant. Some of them seem to need the pacifier for complete oral gratification.

When we first became parents we equipped ourselves with a pacifier along with all the other usual infant paraphernalia. I tried it a few times with Peter and later with Anne when they were fussy and had had what I felt was sufficient milk or juice or cuddling. Both children rejected the pacifier. Joy, on the other hand, had become accustomed to a pacifier during her three lonely months in an orphanage, and she continued to use it occasionally for several months after she joined us. I will not generalize from this that children who accept pacifiers are those who have lacked love and attention. I suggest that parents not allow themselves or their infants to become overly dependent on pacifiers and that they remove them from the scene after the child reaches two.

It is much easier to break the pacifier habit than the thumb-sucking habit. Some dentists believe that persistent thumb-sucking beyond the age of two may aggravate malocclusion of the teeth. If the infant begins thumb sucking, it seems reasonable to transfer that urge to a pacifier, which can be eliminated later on. However, pediatric dentists tell me that if children are forceful suckers on the pacifier it, too, may damage the mouth anatomy even in children under two. On the other hand, children who use the pacifier gently and infrequently may continue to do so indefinitely without injury.

If parents wish to help the child overcome the pacifier habit, it helps if they convince themselves that their child can live happily without it. If they feel they can provide substitutes during the first days of "withdrawal," the cold-turkey approach may be best. Substitutes may include lying down with the child until he is asleep at night, extra play with the child, and after two years, special treats such as Popsicles (made from juice or yogurt), carrot sticks, cucumber strips, cauliflower, apple wedges. Gradual withdrawal of the pacifier may be better for some parents and some children. There's no one way and no easy way. The need for oral gratification obviously persists in many adults and can be manifested by pipe sucking, cigar chomping and gum chewing.

Jealousy

House guests or a new baby or other changes in the home routine can affect small children differently from adults. Peter's reaction when we had a visit from four teen-age cousins and their parents was quite similar to the jealous reaction of some toddlers at the arrival of a new baby in the house.

> August 6—Peter slept poorly, had frequent tantrums and several shrieking episodes during the four-day visit. He messed his pants often during the day, but not once at night. We had intended that he should sleep in his room and share it with his boy cousins. But after the first night he crawled in with us at around 11:00. Despite all the fun and excitement of the guests, his comment when we saw them off today was, "All gone. No come back."

Peter, at age two and a half, was obviously jealous of the extra attention given the house guests and tried to draw more attention to himself by regressing in toilet training and by crying and shrieking. This can seem like a problem to parents, especially if the house guests are in-laws.

Jealousy probably stems from perceiving oneself as threatened by someone or something. Peter may have been threatened by the size of the older cousins and by their athletic skills which he did not yet possess. He most surely was threatened by the loss of attention and tried to recapture some of that by joining us in bed—something he did frequently, but only at get-up times.

Since few people—children or adults—have perfect ego strength and self-assurance, jealously is likely to be noted in most families. Two- and three-year-olds tend to manifest it overtly. They may fear that the new baby is replacing them, perhaps because they were inadequate or not good enough for the satisfaction of their parents. Their overt expression of this fear may not be immediately recognizable as fear. It may appear to be hostility and aggression. When the object of a child's fear or jealousy is a new baby, it is fortunate that the child usually shows his feelings in blatant fashion. This reminds parents to be on the alert for battering problems. Sometimes, although the older child can pretend affection when the parents are around, he may clobber the baby when they're out of sight. What can be done?

Here are some suggestions for helping toddlers who are jealous of baby.

1. Avoid leaving such young siblings together unattended.
2. Stress the "big boy" or "big girl" idea to the older child. Like, "You taught the baby how to walk. He watched you and now he can walk, too." Or, "Are you teaching the baby to talk?"
3. Engage in some activity with the older child which excludes the younger. "You can go shopping with me, but the baby has to stay home. She's too young to go."
4. If guests are focusing on the baby to the exclusion of the older child, direct them to the older child, or cuddle him yourself during those moments.

The same suggestions can be adapted to easing jealousy over house guests or other threatening perceptions in the life of a toddler.

Negativism

The negative streak that lurks in all of us tends to peak in small children at about age two. Here's how it went with our two-and-a-half-year-old:

> August 19—Peter didn't want to go to nursery school this morning and I said, "Never mind." He spent a quiet, placid morning playing with three decrepit toy cars. But at nap time he became very negative. "No" seemed to be the only word he knew.
>
> "Would you like to rest?" "No."
> "Would you like to write?" "No."
> "Would you like to ride your tractor?" "No."
> "Would you like ice cream?" "No."
> There were two minutes of silence. Suddenly he said, "Please, I *want* ice cream." I gave him a big dish, and he settled down.

Negativism is more obvious in vigorous, intensely reacting, "mother-killer"'type children than in quiet, calm, placid children. An obsessive-compulsive, perfectionist parent may find it especially hard to take. It has been a problem with me. But I know that the child is trying to say, "I am a person. I am unique." Simply suppressing the negativism is not a very useful thing to do to a toddler unless the negativism is leading him directly into a dangerous situation, like touching the fire when you said, "Don't touch."

In spite of the "No," young children realize that they are still dependent, and they will more easily acquiesce to a given requirement after the "No" has been permitted. If possible, they should not be exposed to a long succession of situations that give them the opportunity to use "No." For example:

"Anne, I'm going to the store. Want to come along?"

"No, no."

Or if I pick her up and say, "We're going, don't argue with me," Anne will go screaming to the store and neither of us will get what we wanted out of that little trip. But instead, if I calmly put on my coat and head for the door, Anne will likely follow me. After all, she really does like to go along on errands.

In this example, Anne did not really have a choice, and I should not have used the ritual expression "Want to come along?" Negativism can be less bothersome if we do not give many choices to two-year-olds. Questions like "Do you want to go to bed?" and "Do you want some peas?" and "Do you want your bath?" are best avoided. But, "Do you want your ice cream?" and "Do you want to play with this toy?" are questions a two-year-old can answer as he or she wishes.

Sometimes use of the double bind helps to reduce negativism. I believe it to be a technique which many parents learn on their own. Examples of the double bind are, "Would you like to eat your peas on the Melmac or the Noritake China?" "Would you like to eat your carrots with your spoon or Anne's spoon?" "When we go to nursery school, would you like to ride in the front or the back?" "When we're through at the dentist's, would you like to stop at McDonald's or at Gino's?" "Would you like to wear your blue pajamas or your yellow pajamas to bed?"

Negativism doesn't end at age three by any means. Some six-year-olds become very negative as they seek further independence. And no doubt the same negative bent experienced by two-year-olds is felt by most adults when patronizing superiors question us.

Exploration, Dangers and Accidents

Exploration is vital to the normal development and learning processes of toddlers. There is evidence to suggest that the exploratory period between one and two years is the most crucial of all developmental periods, especially with regard to creativity and intelligence.

When children this age do not have the energy to move around and explore new things, they miss an important period of their development.

We should be thankful, therefore, if we have strong healthy toddlers with lots of energy for exploration. But with exploration comes danger and possible accidents, as we discovered during a major family move:

> October 6—The American Express man came to our hotel room with a bill. Daddy was out on an errand, so I went to the door to speak with the man. When I turned back into the room a few minutes later, I saw Peter coming out the closet and saying, "It tastes bad, Mama." I looked, and to my horror, saw him holding the broken pieces of a camphor cake. I was terribly frightened, for I have seen kids die from small amounts of camphor. I berated myself for having no ipecac* in the luggage. For two frantic hours we tried to get emergency medical care in a foreign city. We ended up in the hospital, where they tried to pump Peter's stomach. The doctor couldn't get the tube down. I finally concluded that if Peter had actually ingested any of the camphor, he would surely be dead by now. We went back to the hotel, and he was fine.

Admittedly, free exploration carries dangers with it. Child-

*Syrup of ipecac is a non-prescriptive medicine used to induce vomiting.

ren cannot taste scouring powders and furniture polish or poke screwdrivers into electrical outlets without inviting disaster. Dr. Joel Alpert, a well-known American pediatrician, has done a study which suggests that accidental ingestions by children are not truly "accidental." An angry, upset, anxious household may reflect itself in a pre-schooler who eats iron pills, aspirin—or a camphor cake. In our situation the hotel was strange, my husband and I were consumed with all that "had to be done" before we left the hotel, and Peter undoubtedly picked that up. Dr. Alpert points out that in a typical situation the iron pills may have been available to a searching toddler for many months, but the ingestion occurs when the child is left unexpectedly with a babysitter while the mother is driven to the hospital in premature labor.

Ideally we should neither hinder the right of the child to explore, nor should we trust a child always to be reasonable about exploration. One of the times we hinder exploration is when we rely excessively on TV to hold our children's attention. The U.S. average of 54 hours per week of TV watching for pre-school children is excessive. We also hinder exploration by excessive use of playpens and by structuring too much of our children's play. All these excesses may limit the time a child has for exploration as well as limit his available choices of objects to study. For example, pots, pans, magazines and even daddy's shoes may be better objects for his exploration than the toys that are made and marketed by adults.

While the children explore, and while we do our very best not to inhibit them, they do need to be watched. Reasonable precautions can be taken such as putting safety gates on stairs and safety plugs in electrical outlets. And the close observation that is required to allow an eighteen-month-old toddler to do a maximum of exploration is fatiguing, demanding, and sometimes boring. The same can be said for creating a guarded environment where a four-year-old can practice his independence. These duties are best shared with spouses and with mature babysitters.

Attention Getting and Negativism

The desire to get attention explains much of what we call naughty or destructive behavior in children and helps explain the same manifestations in adults. If your five-year-old is having a birthday party and his friends are just starting to arrive, that's when you can expect to notice an embarrassing smell from your three-year-old who up to that moment was thought to be completely toilet trained. It gets attention. The same result might be achieved with a tantrum in the middle of the living room or a loud rendition of a new song. Regrettably, no attention comes from helping big brother put gift wrapping in the wastebasket as he opens his presents, nor from most of the accepted activities for a younger sibling at a birthday party. Our daughter Anne, at age seventeen months, made an early discovery about attention getting:

> November 28—Anne, who seems to need less attention than the others, has been in a funny stage. It started two weeks ago when we were visiting at the cousins and Peter bumped his head outside. It earned him lots of sympathy from his aunt, and Anne was watching. She then walked over to the same spot, bent over, and very gently banged her own head. My sister understood and lavished Anne with fake solace. This was a marvelous discovery for Anne, and she has been repeating her fake head injury act many times since.
>
> Now as I write, and try to ignore her, she is jabbering more and more loudly . . . "ehhhh" . . . "eeeehhhh" . . .

Attention Getting and Negativism

> "EHHHHHHHH." It means "I want your pen, Mommy," and it means "I want attention, Mommy." I must give her that now, and I put my pen down.

Children do not always differentiate between angry attention and loving attention. So parents must practice giving more attention to positive actions than to negative ones. With practice we can program ourselves to say a kind word about the smiling face, "thank you" for the coat hung up, praise for getting into the car on time.

As we become more spontaneous in our warm comments about positive actions, we can expect our children to make spontaneous positive comments about the behavior of others. As they grow older, they may be influenced by the outside world and the media which seem to give more attention to negative behavior. Hopefully their pre-school programming about attention getting with positive behavior will take precedence over later lessons.

What to do about negative behavior? The easy answer, "Ignore it," certainly isn't always easy to implement. The Transactional Analysis approach—telling your child, "You've hooked my child by acting like that"—may evoke the response "Ha, ha, I've hooked your child." Children learn the current jargon as fast or faster than we. The old cliche "Johnny, I love you, but I don't like what you do" may fail to influence a stormy four-year-old as much as it should; nor does the "You make me feel sad" approach always work.

The apparent immediate trigger of "naughtiness" in a young child does not often warrant prolonged analysis, but parents might ask if they are the models for negativism in their children. Children copy parental speech, gestures, walks, and physical symptoms. They can also imitate negative statements and acts of parents, siblings, playmates, and TV characters.

If we can encourage our children to see themselves as responsible for what they do and for what happens to them, they may find it more difficult to be negative because the object of the negativism must then be themselves. It's much easier to be negative if I believe that everything I don't like is someone else's fault. Of course, in the case of the two-year-old who is not yet blaming anyone, it's best to cuddle him through his yells and not risk having them repressed.

Separation Anxiety

During this period I was with the children nearly all the time except for occasional absences of a few hours. Yet, Anne's need for extra security was obvious:

> December 5—Had a nice day at the Johnsons'. The kids seemed overtired during the trip home, but now at 8 p.m. Anne is still wandering around. She has seemed insecure during the last two nights. Her "Momism" is increasing. She is nearly seventeen months, and I know this is getting near the time when separation anxiety peaks. She is also cutting three teeth, had four loose bowel movements today and sleeps badly. She asks for "bobble" at unusual times. I fear that breaking her away from the bottle is going to be rough. She also asks me to cuddle her at odd moments.

Separation anxiety, the fear an infant experiences when he is away from mother or principal caretaker, is usually observed initially at seven or eight months and peaks around twenty months.

It is a normal part of development as the dependent infant recognizes his own being and that of others. Psychology attaches much significance to this period and its effect on adult life. Pediatricians look for separation anxiety during well-baby examinations and recognize developmental lag and sometimes emotional deprivation if its early signs do not appear by the end of the first year.

The innate personality of the baby affects his manifestation of separation anxiety. Infants who react maximally to all stresses from birth may do so later on when they are anxious about separation from principal caretakers. They may show their fear and anxiety by screaming, kicking and hitting. Other infants have the same fears with less outward manifestations. They may not eat when their mother is gone, or they eat excessively; or they do not sleep, or they sleep all the time. Many mothers have said to me, "He sleeps all day with the babysitter and really comes to life when I return; he won't sleep for me."

Separation anxiety, although normal as defined, may be increased or prolonged by anxieties or fears of parents over what might happen when they are away from the infant or toddler. The young child can perceive these and may reflect more anxiety. I am not a proponent of ad-lib absences of parents from their children. But separation of children from parents eventually occurs in most families, and the path for both the toddler and the parents can be smoothed in several ways:

1. Infants should be left with babysitters occasionally during the periods when they are awake during their early months.

2. If both parents plan to work outside the home and leave their baby with someone who is not a usual member of the household, this preferably should be arranged before six to seven months of age or after two years. A child who has never been left with a stranger and is suddenly separated from parents at the age of eighteen months may be severely

traumatized.

3. Parents should express warmth and hospitality toward visitors in the home. Young babies will recognize that other humans are liked and accepted by their parents and will be more likely to do likewise with babysitters.

4. Babies should be exposed to the sights and sounds of the culture and society in which the parents live.

In primitive societies infants do not stay with one exclusive caretaker during their first two years. Relatives and friends and older children in villages will act as parent surrogates. This makes emotional trauma less likely if the parents are removed.

I have seen emotionally traumatized two-year-olds who were abruptly thrust into the care of strangers when parents had to be hospitalized. If possible, infants should be prepared for such contingencies. Recently one of our neighbors called in a panic because she had just received a call from police that her husband had been injured and taken to a nearby hospital. She asked my husband to drive her to the hospital. I ran to her house to get the children—ages fifteen months, four years, eight years, and nine years. I recall the frightened look on her face as she ran for our car thrusting the fifteen-month-old baby boy towards me. I knew the older children, but I had not seen the baby before. As his mother rushed off he burst into frightened screams, and I could not calm him. The older children were also crying. I soothed them and then put the baby in the arms of his nine-year-old brother, where he quieted. The separation lasted for two hours, and the father was not seriously injured. The baby boy chortled as he saw his mother reappear. Two hours of such trauma will probably not cause lasting scars—two weeks might.

Separation anxiety wanes after twenty-four months, and normal children usually separate easily from their mothers at least for brief periods by three years. Pediatricians watch for that, too. But separation anxiety may recur at various times of stress or fatigue, and many college freshmen or military recruits have a twinge of it when they find themselves outside the family nest.

Eating Habits

No country in the world has so great a variety of foods or of eating habits as does the United States. Pediatricians probably answer more questions about eating than about any other behavior problems of children.

> December 8—I am impressed by the amount of food the kids consume. Peter eats huge quantities for breakfast, which is likely to include eggs, four or five pieces of toast, two cups of milk. He also likes yogurt. We feed the children on a very regular schedule, and I am convinced that each eats more in a day than I. Here's their average daily diet:

	Joy (11 months)	Peter and Anne (3 years) (17 months)
Breakfast	Rice Pablum and fruit Yogurt	Oatmeal or eggs Toast Pancakes (occasionally)
10:00 a.m.	Apple juice	Apple juice Graham crackers
11:30 a.m.	Rice, pureed beef and vegetable Milk	Rice, chopped meat and vegetable Milk
2:30 p.m.	Crackers	Crackers Yogurt or milk

5:00 p.m.	Rice, pureed beef and vegetable	Rice plus chopped meat and vegetables or potatoes Occasional dessert (once a week on the average)

Peter drinks 2-3 cups of whole milk per day.
Anne drinks 16-20 ounces of skim milk per day.
Joy drinks 24-32 ounces of skim milk per day.

The average child gains fifteen pounds in the first year of life, and four to six pounds per year thereafter until age six or seven. It seems logical that his food intake decreases in the second year, but not so to many parents. Thus, children are overfed and develop neuroses over meal times. The pattern for subsequent obesity and related cardiovascular disease may be set by excessive fats and sweets consumed by infants and toddlers.

In spite of studies which claim that two-year-olds will naturally choose a balanced diet if given free access to a variety of foods, I have begun to wonder why children, even young children, seem to prefer a diet which is not ideal. Are they imitating their role models, or is it instinctive to prefer hot dogs, catsup, potato chips, milk shakes, soft drinks and sugared breakfast cereal to cooked breakfast cereal, fish, vegetables and fruits? Surely they will eat some of the last-mentioned foods if that is all that's available. In our household we try, with some success, to live by a rule of no sugared cereals, no candy, no cookies and no potato chips. Yet the children often clamor to eat at fast hamburger restaurants. Therefore, with partial tongue in cheek I offer the following suggestions:

1. Do not force a child to eat. (We broke this rule.)
2. Expect a reduction of appetite after the first year of life.
3. Emphasize a nutritious breakfast containing non-

sugared cereals, occasional eggs, juice and milk. I have heard many mothers say, "It's such a hassle in the morning. I've given up trying to get nutritious food into them. I figure it's better to get something in them even if it is 'Crispy Sweets'." *Bad breakfast food should not be in the house.* For the hard-to-please child, one might try whole grain toast with peanut butter, yogurt, fruits or various cheeses.

4. Avoid serving sugary snacks. We suggest fruits, carrot sticks, celery sticks, nuts or raisins. Raisins, however, are not recommended by some pedodontists, for they stick to teeth. If your child must have cookies, make them from nutritious ingredients, minimizing sugar content. There are many cookbooks which contain recipes for nutritious cookies.

5. Sandwiches are traditional for American pre-schoolers at lunch time. Nutritious sandwiches can be made if whole grain breads are used along with meats, cheeses, lettuce, cucumbers, tuna, tomatoes, sardines, kippers, etc., instead of the sugar, jellies and jam which children prefer.

6. Avoid serving sweet desserts routinely. Children are bound to receive excess sweets at times. There are birthday parties, nursery school snacks, doting grandparents and generous neighbors who see to that.

7. Use skim or two percent milk instead of whole milk beyond age two. Avoid powdered soft drinks and carbonated beverages. Water is a fine drink.

8. Remember that the easiest way to keep a child eating the right foods is to keep the wrong foods out of the house. If parents like to snack on Danish pastries, doughnuts, potato chips and cola drinks, they cannot expect more from their child.

9. Avoid using sweets as a reward.

Toilet Training

During the year that we had three in diapers at one time, we were just beginning to learn to use our imaginations to anticipate an outcome like the wonderful day when the diapers and training pants were no longer necessary. It helped to keep us moderately sane. When Peter was almost three and Anne was seventeen months, I wrote:

> December 14—Peter tries to shape houses, cats, rivers in the sand, and Anne destroys them. For the last two days Anne has been interested in her potty again, and uses it often for urinating.
>
> A few days ago when Peter was denied a wish by Daddy, he became furious. He stood and fussed for a few seconds, ran out on the porch, and returned a few minutes later to announce, "My pants are wet." We ignored the statement. Shortly thereafter he shucked his pants, went to the bathroom and, a few minutes later, announced proudly that he had gone poo-poo in the toilet.

As many mothers know, child psychologists suggest restraint for parents who are inclined to push toilet training. It is easy for me to parrot their advice. "You'll know when he's ready." "Don't express displeasure if he has an accident." "Set her on the potty chair several times a day and let her get accustomed to it." "Be patient."

Intellectually, I know that restraint is good advice. But I also know that mothers get frustrated and angry over wet spots on upholstery, stool spilled on rugs or in bathwater, the piles of dirty diapers and training pants and wet sheets. If a mother spanks a three-year-old found sitting in his stool—or, as I heard of one doing, batting stool around the room with a tennis racket—she feels guilty. Grandparents are notoriously forgetful in this regard and are no help when they insist that the long-suffering mother was completely trained at eight months!

As a practical matter, it is not possible to recommend a single toilet training routine which is applicable to every child. It helps if all members of a household can agree on an approach to toilet training and reinforce the principal caretaker. If Daddy could not care less and lets Johnny run around in messy pants while Mommy is out shopping, Johnny will be less motivated to use the potty chair.

Consider that:

1. Bowel control comes naturally before bladder control.
2. In spite of what others say, most children are not reliable about daytime bladder control until three to four years.
3. Some children fear the commode and should not be forced on it.
4. Habitual stool retention might be triggered by a parent who is too aggressive in promoting bowel control. Daily elimination may not be necessary for everyone.
5. Bed-wetting should not be a concern until the child is five-and-a-half years.
6. Wet pants, messed pants and wet beds may be attention-getting devices. Praise for positive things the child does instead of condemnation for wet pants may reduce the number of wet pants.
7. At the start of toilet training, a potty chair can be placed in the bathroom for the child to use sometime after he reaches one year. This will make it a familiar object. If the child sits on the chair occasionally with all clothing on, no rush should be made to disrobe him. When he begins to have bowel movements at regular times (and this may not happen until age two), the parents can begin to place the child on the potty chair with his diaper off. If this meets with resistance or fear, parents should hold off a few days or weeks and try again.

When the toddler is fortunate enough to have a bowel movement while sitting on the potty, praise him—but not excessively. Do not flush the produce immediately or in the child's presence until parents are convinced that all is going well. The toddler may get the message about bowel movements after his first success, or after many. Sooner or later every human of normal intelligence and physiology becomes toilet trained.

Nighttime Waking and Crying

Toward the end of this diary year, we moved into our new home in a new city after several months of travel, staying with relatives and at hotels and a beach cottage.

> December 26—The children are now back to their regular living schedules and seem quite content, even though all of them—plus their parents—have upper respiratory infections. During the first night Joy began one of her nighttime crying jags. We were so beat I said to Daddy, "We're in our own place. Joy is in her own room. Relatives and neighbors aren't listening. I'll look to see if she's all right and, if so, let her go to sleep on her own." Daddy objected, but I insisted. Six months of getting up to assuage her wails was enough, and I was really tired. So she cried for about twenty minutes, went to sleep, and hasn't bothered us at night for four nights. Nor have Peter and Anne come traipsing into their parents' bedroom in the middle of the night. I guess they sense that we are home again.

Many infants will sleep through the night, i.e., eight to ten consecutive hours by age two months. Parents may then enjoy uninterrupted nights of sleep (unless they also happen to have a toddler who is awakening with frightening dreams) until the infant is about six or eight months. At that time, waking associated with crying may recur. This might be triggered by illness or teething or some family disruption, but it also seems to be a normal part of the development which coincides with further maturation of the brain and perhaps the beginning of separation anxiety.

If this waking is reinforced with rocking, walking, extra feedings, it may go on for months or years. Parents who have only one child may be able to do this and enjoy it. Parents who have several children and/or the requirement to arise early each morning may become tired and irritable as a result of the nightly interruptions. Then nocturnal waking and crying is a problem, and something should be done about it.

Some parents solve it by taking the infant into bed with them. This may allow all to sleep if the infant is not the type who regards 3 a.m. as a special time for play. The inclination of sleepy parents to sleep with the child is not necessarily bad, although the professors of psychiatry whom I heeded during my training suggested that this would lead to sexual problems. For many years I was convinced that it was wrong for children to sleep with their parents. Then during the first month of breast feeding Anne, when I was very tired and she awakened for her 2 a.m. feeding, I found it more natural and comfortable to take her into our bed for nursing. Theory flew out the window in the face of my early-morning fatigue.

Time may prove that children develop more securely when allowed in bed with their parents. Personally, I don't sleep well with too many in the bed; but the 2 a.m. cuddling, the going to sleep routine with parent lying beside child, and the good morning entrances of children into bed with parents all seem to be happy times. I recognize that there has been only one year of my life when I have not shared a bed or bedroom with a sibling, a college roommate or my husband; so, not surprisingly, I don't like sleeping alone.

Our diary indicates that all our children have been in and out of each others' or our beds for years; but not for all night, except when one or the other of the children has been very ill. I prefer to sleep with a young child who has a high fever or croup or vomiting illness. With time the entrances of our children into our bed have become more rare and usually occur when they awaken in the morning.

Back to Joy's nightly wakings. Her problem (or mine) was not being solved by taking her into our bed. She was a restless sleeper. Allowing her to "cry it out" was successful. The expectation of parents that this will work is probably crucial to its success. Here again it's important to look for the light at the end of the tunnel.

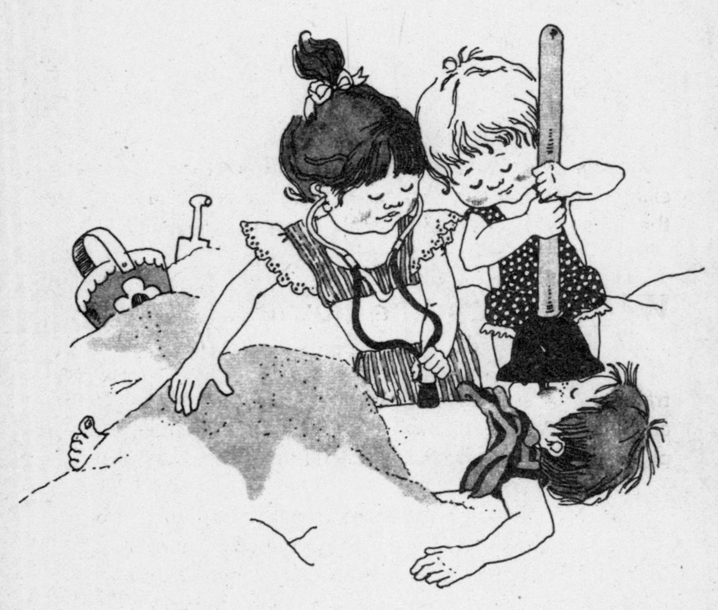

Creativity in children . . . makes them frightfully busy, messy, and happy.

2
Life with children aged one to four

As the year started, Peter had just turned three, Anne was eighteen months, Joy was celebrating her first birthday, and the family had settled into a new home in a new city.

Weaning from the Bottle

Weaning is sometimes very easy and sometimes a very traumatic process for both the parents and the baby. In the case of Anne, it happened accidentally. In an earlier entry I programmed weaning to be difficult for Anne. I was wrong!

> January 5—Last night I forgot to fix a bedtime "bobble" for Anne. So did she. It happened again tonight. She did not comment on its absence. I think she is over the bottle and out of diapers at eighteen months.

To give a broader view of our family experience with weaning, I will break from the chronology of the diary to pick up an entry more than three years later when Anne was five and Joy was four. I had promised each of the girls a bedtime story about themselves when they were babies. Anne asked for a story about her first birthday party. Joy asked about her baby bottle.

Weaning from the Bottle

(Three years later)—I told how Joy had loved her bottle as an infant until she was nearly two, and then began biting off the nipples when she was given her bedtime bottle. She soon used up all her nipples; and each time I would need to come in and change her pajamas and sheets, which were soaked with milk. Thus she came to the end of her bottles.

Joy said, "I didn't want to hear that. I didn't do that."

I then talked about Anne and how she had started tossing her bottles out of the crib shortly before she stopped asking for them. Anne said, "I didn't want them anyway, Mommy."

When the stories were over, Anne went to sleep immediately. Joy was thrashing around in her bed for a while; and after the room became quiet, I thought she was asleep. Around 10:00 she came out and said, "What you told me made tears come out of my eyes. About not giving us any more bottles. Why did you do that?"

Joy and Anne illustrate the common observation that the bottle is much more important to some children than it is to others. Joy had kept her bottle habit longer than do many toddlers. I was hesitant to deny the bottle because her early orphanage experience had made her unusually dependent on it for comfort. So she was allowed a bedtime bottle for several months after daytime bottles had been replaced by cups of liquid.

I was always careful, however, to remove the bottle after she was asleep. Children's dentists point out that a bottle partly filled with juice or milk which can dribble into the baby's mouth intermittently throughout the night is disastrous for the front teeth in particular. Water is a better bottle drink at sleep time. And, from the perspective of a pediatrician, I was concerned about choking and aspiration if a sleepy baby decided to suck from the bottle in the middle of the night.

In spite of Joy's retrospective bemoaning, the diaries do not indicate that weaning was a problem in our family. We were not rigid about time schedules. We simply expected that our children would learn to drink from cups before they reached nursery-school age. And they did.

While editing this chapter I thought it would be interesting to refresh the girls' memories with respect to their weaning. They were now eight. So while we were loading the dishwasher, I said, "Boy, it's sure been a long time since I've washed any baby bottles. Do you girls remember when we stopped using the bottles?" Joy replied, "No, but didn't I throw my bottle out of the bed?" I said, "No that wasn't you, that was Anne. Do you remember what you did?" "No." Joy was losing interest in the conversation. I went on, "You bit off the top of your nipples." Her eyes lit up. "Did I get a milk shampoo? Hey, Anne, I had a milk shampoo when I was a baby." End of conversation.

The decision about when to give up the bottle should take into account the wishes of the baby as well as those of parents and pediatricians. If parents consider it important that a baby be weaned by a specific age—for example, at eighteen months—then it is probably easier to have the baby go through weaning then to have the parents worry about it.

One reason why some babies continue to demand their bottle may be that their caretakers rely excessively on the bottle as a way to occupy or soothe the baby. It may be easier to fill a bottle and pop it in the baby's mouth than to prepare solid foods or help them hold a cup. The disease known as iron deficiency anemia has been associated with the excessive use of non-iron-fortified milk-filled bottles for infants and toddlers.

Weaning from the Bottle

A dangerous extreme of using a bottle for the convenience of parents was demonstrated by the mother of one of my patients who would leave her eight-month-old alone in the apartment while she went shopping for several hours. She placed the baby in a playpen with three eight-ounce bottles of milk placed around the edges. When she returned, all the bottles would be empty and the baby asleep.

Prepare early for weaning, whether from the bottle or the breast:

1. Offer liquids from a cup beginning at age five or six months.
2. Stop offering midnight feedings after the baby is two or three months old and is able to sleep through the night.
3. Avoid use of the bottle as a soporific at times when the parents want the baby quiet.
4. Wean breast-fed babies directly from breast to cup as soon as the baby is old enough to manage a cup.

How do you know when the baby is ready to give up the bottle? When you offer liquid in a cup and the baby drinks well. Or when the bottle is not in sight, and he doesn't clamor for it. Or when he is put to bed with the bottle and immediately throws it out. Or when he bites off the nipple and dumps the milk out. We can accept such clues as meaning that the baby has weaned himself.

Early Waking

Infants and children, like their parents, have sleep cycles which vary in the numbers of hours of sleep required as well as in the preferred time of day or night for sleeping. Some babies sleep twenty out of twenty-four hours during the early months. Others need only a maximum of twelve hours sleep in a day. Some like to go to bed late and wake late. Others are the opposite.

Even parents who have an "early to bed, early to rise" cycle may have days when they like to sleep late. That is rarely possible A.C. (after children).

February 2 and 7—Peter and Anne came pattering into bed around 5 a.m. Peter often joins us around this time. He is in the nude, having carefully removed his wet pajamas before getting into bed with us.

Even a late-sleeping baby or toddler is likely to be awake by 7 a.m. This may be a clue that here is a child who will later sleep through the school bus. Early-waking children are usually up between five and six. Fortunately, they are often in good humor at this time. The inclination of most of them is to jump into bed with their parents.

After ten years of those early morning intrusions, we still find ourselves unable to resist them. Eventually this very special time will end. Some parents may be unable to tolerate such early morning entrances because of their own sleep habits and needs. And if the children are not allowed to enter their parents' bed in the morning, I believe parents should be gentle in telling them so. Also, toddlers should not be allowed to roam the house unsupervised for very long during those early morning hours.

First Questions about Sex

Questions about sex come early and are normal and innocent. Peter was a little over three years old when he noticed a difference between the sexes.

March 2—It is Sunday evening, and I have done only babysitting this weekend. The children have been

> quite good-humored. Yesterday Peter and Anne went shopping with Daddy. Last night we put a fire in the fireplace, and the kids enjoyed it. We are allowing Joy to eat with her spoon and fingers and she enjoys her own mess. I worry because she continues to put dirt, stones and toys in her mouth.
>
> Peter noted that Anne was not able to urinate while standing and asked me where her penis was. I explained that she was a girl and never had a penis. He asked me if I had one . . . if Mary did . . . if Daddy did . . . and he seemed happy with the answers.

When a toddler asks where babysitter's penis is, he should be answered frankly and at his intellectual level. He need not be told the mechanism of intercourse. When a three-year-old insists adamantly that she was never inside mommy's tummy, there is no need for argument—just as when later on she will likely say that only she and she alone was in mommy's tummy.

Toddlers inspect each others' genitalia. There is nothing to be gained by preventing siblings from looking at each other. Current books, magazines, television shows and radio programs stress the importance of early sex education done by parents; but the average parent (no matter how educated, sophisticated, promiscuous) has a moment of panic each time a six- or seven-year-old says, "What does F-U-C-K mean? It was written on our bus today." Or, "David used that word in class today." This crucial moment is evaded by many of today's "enlightened" parents. At the moment of truth they fall flat. They pretend the problem will go away. It does, for the child finds another way to get his answer.

Parents, probably because of the way they learned about sexuality themselves, are reluctant to admit to their children that they have had sexual intercourse. Children nonetheless follow through with very direct, explicit questions.

"What does it feel like, Daddy?"

One of my patient's parents reported that their seven-year-old boy had asked, "Do you bite Mama's neck the way a rooster does?"

No one can tell a child about sex better than his parents. Children are going to learn amazingly early from us or from other informers. When they ask their parents, they should be answered truthfully.

Linguistic Precision

I continue to be surprised by the number of bright school children I see who lack correct terms for sex and execretory functions. Toddlers might have difficulty with words like "urinate" or "defecate," but can easily say words such as "pee" and "poop"; so it is easy to understand how these become the common terms. However, I have found that some families seem not even to have a common vernacular word for urinate. They may refer euphemistically to "going to the bathroom"—or simply "bathroom" or "draining" or "go potty"—without distinguishing urination from defecation. We believed it important for our children to know the correct words. In my wisdom I went one better.

> March 4—Peter came home from nursery school in his usual high spirits. While we were enjoying lunch he suddenly said, "Mama, I told the teacher I had to leave to micturate, and she didn't know what I meant." I roared. Peter roared. I suggested he use the word "urinate" in the future.

Early Memory

Children amaze us from time to time by recalling specific details of what occurred in their second or third year of life. Peter was three months past his third birthday when I wrote:

> March 10—Peter often gives evidence of having a good memory. Last night he said, "Did I take Heather and go for a walk down the road to see the trucks, Mama? And was Aunt Barbara afraid we would be run over by a truck?" He was right. This event had occurred six months ago, and I had forgotten it until he reminded me.

Most likely, children will not consciously recall events like these at age fifteen or twenty. But the fact of conscious memory at ages three to six or seven or even later for events which occurred in the infancy and toddler stage should make parents more aware of our importance as models during the first years of a child's life.

Events and observations made by very young children are incorporated into their belief systems for a lifetime. Conscious memories and beliefs become subconscious memories and beliefs which are incorporated into adult conscious beliefs and behavior. And the beliefs of toddlers may be based on faulty interpretations.

Children interpret conversations, songs, stories and poems with a more limited vocabulary and more concrete understanding than adults do. If we listen carefully to toddlers we often hear evidence of this and sometimes it makes us laugh. For instance, eight months later I recorded:

> After dinner Daddy was lying on Anne's bed as the children were playing nearby. He called out to me,

"I've got something on my mind I've got to tell you, but I've forgotten what it is." Immediately Anne ran to him, stared carefully at all aspects of his head and said, finally, "Where is it Daddy?" She was twenty-eight months old. She was looking for "something."

I recall from my own childhood my complete confusion over the meaning of Christmas carols which I had memorized after hearing them before I could read. And I remember my horror over the phrase "to fire" an employee, thinking that a person fired was literally ignited.

Children may appear to comprehend a statement, but the comprehension may be based on limited vocabularies and definitions for the many words in our language which sound alike. Hence a six-year-old asks, "What is the stock market—is that where you buy cows?"

Young children also interpret stories, movies and television programs concretely and cannot always differentiate what is real and what is pretend. They will weep over "Snow White" or panic over "Jack and the Beanstalk" or yell furiously at a cruel schoolmaster in "Little House on the Prairie." Since watching television and movies may place them in a hyper-suggestible state, interpretations and beliefs, both useful and harmful, may imprint their subconscious minds—perhaps forever. This is an area that is just being recognized as an important one to study. Parents can help by watching television with their children. They can point out the concept of pretend, ask them what they think happened and, when children are older, discuss the merits of the program.

Toilet Logistics

Some diary entries defy categorizing. The following is—so help me—a verbatim quote from the diary. I even gave it a title, "89th in a Series on the Joys of Motherhood." I remember that later I was amused enough to send a copy to my mother. At the time I was not.

> April 8—Yesterday afternoon we returned from a vacation weekend. Everyone was a little tired and sunburned, and I wasn't much in the mood to consider excretory problems of the children. In fact I rejoiced over the fact that we had driven for two hours without an interruption resulting from the accumulation of solid wastes.
>
> I had just started making supper for the children and Daddy had gone off on an errand when the trouble began. Joy suddenly said, "poo-poo." Since she is not potty trained, any indication from her of comprehension of bowel processes is met with wild enthusiasm by me. I rushed her upstairs to sit on the potty chair and found that she had just barely begun. I removed her diaper, set it aside, and pushed a book under her nose so that her attention might be held while she sat on the potty. Peter was yelling from downstairs. "Anne is sitting on the pot down here, Mama."
>
> "Well, let her sit," I replied. "I am busy with Joy."
>
> Not five seconds later I heard the laborious steps of the little lady ascending. She popped into my bedroom with a broad grin and stuck the pot under my nose. Peter was just behind. I placed the pot in his not-too-dependable hands and said, "I must watch Joy on her potty. You empty this please."
>
> Peter cheerfuly acquiesced; but, a few seconds later he yelled, "Mama, I need a spoon to get it out."
>
> As I groaned, I noted Anne looking uncomfortable and beheld some forgotten pieces falling onto the

floor.

"Peter, bring that pot back, quick," I yelled.

Anne resumed her place, but now Joy was getting restless and had produced nothing. I was feeling a little disjointed and thinking that there was some merit in diapers.

I took Joy to the bathroom which adjoins the children's bedroom, leaving Anne sitting. Anne, with her penchant for independent action, should never be left in such a situation. I cleaned Joy, rinsed her diaper and was replacing it with a clean one when Peter yelled, "Anne is in your bathroom, Mama."

"What is she doing?"

"She's cleaning her potty."

Now I have dealt with stool in trains, on planes, in restaurants, etc.—even at christenings (Anne's); but this was the be-all, end-all. Anne had emptied the potty, all right. Some of it had reached the toilet bowl, but she had also covered the bathroom floor, sink, etc.

Fortunately, Daddy arrived home to watch Joy while I watched Anne and then got out the Lysol bottle for the bathroom. It took me thirty minutes. Cleaning a diaper takes two minutes.

Identification with Parents

Normal children feel that parents are omniscient and omnipotent through their early years. Then as independence increases, horizons widen and some disillusionment sets in, they may find some faults in their parents. This helps set the stage for the eventual separation. However, it is generally agreed that a firm early identification with a father and a mother helps to promote appropriate sex role identification and good ego strength, and eases the eventual separation process.

> April 20—This morning I took the children to the arboretum for two hours. We noted ants, a mouse, a horned lizard and a caterpillar. While we were looking at a very tall tree, Peter exclaimed, "That tree is almost as long as Daddy!" He often talks about getting big like Daddy; and he also says to me, "Mama, when you get big, you can drive Daddy's jeep."

In American culture it has been easier for children to identify with mothers than with fathers. A working pattern which keeps fathers out of homes and inaccessible to their children from dawn until dusk, and homes in which the mother is raising the children alone are primarily responsible for this. Children may find it difficult to understand fathers because they do not see them at work and cannot share their working experiences, as they could when fathers worked on farms or in small towns. (As more mothers continue full-time professions outside the home, children also find it difficult to identify with mothers.) They may see fathers only during times when the fathers are trying to relax, and may develop a mental image of their fathers as crabby people who do not want to listen to children while sipping beer or watching television at night; or, on the other hand, as the people who do all the fun things with children while mommies grow irritable in their preoccupation with household chores. The plural is used because a child is likely to project his image of his father and his mother to other fathers and mothers. Neither the view of fathers as remote and crabby people nor as providers of constant fun is likely to prepare a boy or girl for a happy adult life.

Identification with Parents

Many children see too much of their mothers or female surrogates during pre-school years and too little of their fathers. Mothers make the majority of day-to-day decisions concerning activities of children and also set discipline patterns. A father's decision to take the family to the beach for a two-week holiday, or to put a four-year-old in a special nursery school, is probably minor in overall effect when compared with the myriad of decisions which a mother normally makes in a year. Mothers or fathers can get fatigued or bored by too many fourteen-hour days of child care, and they may break down as good models. They may recognize their self-importance as existing primarily in relationship to the dependence of their young children. This is fine while the children are young. As the children mature, parents—especially primary caretakers of the children—must find new reasons for living. Otherwise, with our longer life span, the self-image deteriorates and the stage is set for unhappy middle and late years.

For a more natural and healthy identification of children with parents (and vice versa), I suggest the following:

1. Husband and wife should ask themselves before pregnancy: Do we like children? Do we know what they're like? Is one of us willing to give himself or herself to their rearing, especially during the pre-school years? If there are negative answers, it may be better to have no children. This is not a crime. It is an honest, acceptable choice.

2. From infancy on, children should have the opportunity to observe both parents at work and at play.

3. Fathers should spend more of their children's waking hours at home, especially during the initial five or six years. If the mother is the primary wage earner outside of the home, she should endeavor to do the same.

4. Mothers and fathers should not stay with their children beyond points of tolerance, kindness and love. Beyond this point the caretaking must be shared with the other parent

or surrogate parents.

5. Once again, parents should be aware of their roles as models who are observed as they laugh, cry, quarrel, give, take, work, play, lie, etc. Children are masters of taking note of inconsistencies between what parents say and what they do.

6. As a society we should encourage more men to work in day care centers and in nurseries, and also to become primary school teachers.

Real Life in Play

Much of play activity is as true to adult life as the children know how to make it. They want to imitate adults, and this is what they attempt to do.

> April 11—Yesterday Daddy built a house out of packing crates for the kids. How thrilled they were! I made the mistake of saying, "This little room must be the bathroom." So Anne immediately voided in it.

Many, many times I have heard one of my children yelling, "Mama, Mama," and when I respond, the answer is, "No, not you. I want the little Mama." They are involved once again in play acting. They cook, eat, buy, sell, travel, work, laugh and quarrel as they act out family roles. If the real parents give young children opportunities to do real adult things, how delighted they are. Happily, they will buy milk, scrub chairs, stir soup, wash dishes, weed gardens, sew buttons, dust furniture and hammer nails. Unfortunately, somewhere along the line they perceive parental disenchantment with some of these tasks. Thus a two-year-old sweeps with delight; an eight-year-old with reluctance.

I have watched children scolding dolls and stuffed animals,

toilet training them, loving them, giving them medicine and baths.

> April 15—Norwegian Dolly was very special. She stayed on a shelf in her beautiful costume, and she was much admired by the children. She isn't the same any more. After much pleading from Anne, I took "Weegin Dolly" down and placed her in Anne's arms. "She is very special. Take good care of her." I left Anne sitting in a rocker cuddling the doll, and I ran a tub for Peter. I was out of the bathroom no more than two minutes getting Peter. When we returned, "Weegin Dolly," in full costume, was being tenderly bathed.

Play therapy in child psychiatry offers a multitude of objects which the child may use to demonstrate feelings and work out problems. Children also do this in their homes and nursery schools. Parents can learn a great deal by quietly watching children at play.

Biting

During the second and third years of life, children not infrequently use biting to express displeasure or dislike. We experienced it on a not-too-sunny day when Peter was three, Anne was going on two, and Joy sixteen months.

> April 28—Joy cried the whole morning and hit out at anyone who came near her. Her ears looked better, so I couldn't figure out what was upsetting her. Anne had several brief tantrums. Peter came home from nursery school with face and neck wounds and said a bigger boy had bitten him. He denied that he had

attacked first. I wonder what happened?

Some mothers have told me that the cure to biting is to bite the biting child back in order to make him know how it feels. This is a bad example from a prime model and should not be done. Initial biting efforts of a child do not mean that he is aggressive, violent or mean, or that he has a problem. It is likely that human skin falls in the category of teething rings, blocks, spoons, blankets, plastic toys, Daddy's tie or Mother's bracelet to an exploring one- or two-year-old child. What does skin taste like? What is it?

If the exploratory biting efforts are followed by natural signs of distress by the bitten one, it is possible that the toddler will be less inclined to try again. If he gets a bite in return, he may interpret this to mean that bigger people can bite smaller ones and that he has permission to do likewise at his next opportunity.

Perhaps the best way to handle biting is to remove the biter from the play site with gentleness, but saying clearly that he cannot be allowed to play with them again that day. Hopefully the biter soon learns that biting is socially unacceptable.

Bedtime Ritual

Bedtimes should be peaceful, pleasant times. When there are several young children in a household, this may be the way it seems to parents or their offspring. My diary has many entries like the following, made when Anne was twenty-two months old.

> May 5—Peter always asks me to sing at bedtime, but Anne resists the idea by saying loudly, "No, no song," and kicking her legs in disapproval. I wonder why she dislikes my singing so much.

> Her goings-on before she falls asleep are bewildering to me. She lies down a few seconds; then says, "Wee-wee." I say, "Oh, you can go by yourself."
> Sometimes she gets up and goes to the bathroom, and at other times she merely removes her underpants. Then she says, "Blankie, blankie," (meaning blanket) and I put the blanket on her once more. She immediately throws the blanket off when I leave and repeats, "Blankie, blankie."

Parents tend to rush bedtime for their children because of their yearning and need for some quiet time for themselves. The children recognize that. They may feel unwanted and insecure, and so they cry or scream or think of a long list of unfinished business:
"I need a drink."
"I have to go wee-wee."
"My blankets are on wrong."
"Open the door."
"Mama, I have to tell you something."
"I need a Band-Aid."

I suspect that we were similar to many parents in our lack of preparation for the bedtime stunts. As young infants the children went to sleep quite readily at appropriate bedtimes, and we thought that should continue.

The best solution for us was to "join 'em." This might not be the solution for some families, depending on the number and ages of children. With three children who were very close in age and very capable of inciting or stimulating each other to more bedtime high-jinks, we eliminated the problem by lying down with our toddlers until they fell asleep. This was calming to them and to us. We often sang songs or told stories. Two months later in the diary, when Peter was three-and-a-half, I recorded this entry:

Bedtime Ritual

> Peter talked to me about many things while falling asleep. We closed our eyes and told each other what we could see—flowers, animals, etc. Peter said once, "I see it's raining. Can you see it raining, Mama?" A short while later he said, "I see a man on a motorcycle. Now he fell off and the motorcycle's going by itself." And he laughed.
>
> "I see Tobias—two Tobiases—and his little brother."
>
> Such an imagination he has!

As they grew older the children requested specific stories. Sometimes I made them up to contain characters who were like our children. My husband told future stories about what each child might be doing at six or eight or ten. They loved these. If the children seemed excited after an especially active day, I would invite them to use their vivid imaginations and would take a trip through a fairyland playground which culminated with a soft, soft bed that contained pretty sheets and pillows. At that point my darlings would be asleep.

Such bedtimes are a pleasure to recall. When we skipped singing or story telling, we regretted it. Nowadays we try to arrange a family get-together in the living room at night. Each child and parent describes "something good that happened today." We then discuss small concerns. My husband and I tuck the children in and exchange kisses and hugs with them. Sometimes we spend extra time in quiet talk with a child who seems to need it (the phrase in our house is "Mama, can I have a good-night-time?"); and he goes to sleep quickly and peacefully. Insomnia for the children seems to occur only if they have had a cola beverage within a few hours of bedtime.

Tattletales

Tattletaling occurs frequently in situations where children are relating to each other and vying for attention and favor. It begins amazingly early. My daughters were only sixteen and twenty-two months when I became aware that Anne was capable of telling tales.

> May 11—Yesterday the children and I were alone at home. Daddy was out of town. I tried different sorts of amusements for the girls. For a while Anne and Joy were greatly absorbed in pulling cardboard boxes with strings I had attached. They fought intermittently, of course. At 11:30 we walked to the nursery school to fetch Peter. After lunch the children napped from 12:30 to 1:30. While I was putting Peter in the tub before bed, I thought the girls were safely upstairs with me; however, the upstairs gate had been opened, and suddenly I heard Anne's voice coming from the bottom of the stairway. Joy, too, was near the bottom step.
>
> Anne said, "Joy puss me. Joy puss me."
>
> Joy immediately looked at Anne and whispered "Shhh, shhhhhh."
>
> I suspect she may have pushed Anne, but it was amusing to see her trying to curtail the tattletale at sixteen months.

Do the tattlers of early childhood become the gossips of adult years? Is tattling a problem? Parents certainly get tired of it, and this may be good. It discourages children from getting in the habit of saying negative things about others. Daddy will often counter with, "Now tell me something nice about her—I don't want to hear about bad things." Sometimes the accuser will then make a positive statement about the sibling.

More usually the request merely abbreviates or stops the tattling.

The Four-Year-Old

In the turmoil of a house full of small kids there was usually at least one child whose behavior typified one of the traditional stages in child development as described in the Gesell child development books. All children have one thing in common: each is unique and variable, and this tends to confound the experts. We believe that we experienced the "four-year-old" in Peter when he was three-and-half. At the time, Anne had just turned two, and Joy was eighteen months old.

> July 14—As I write Peter is still napping, dirty and disheveled in the playroom where he went to sleep on his own, angry over something.
>
> Peter's imagination is working overtime these days. He converts our hand mixer into a VW bus. Chairs become cars or trains. The other night we awakened to his agonized screeching. He insisted that there was a dog upstairs. His favorite phrase is an emphatic, "But I want to." At times he is very silly, and at times loves to defy me. At other times he says sweetly, "Mama, cuddle me." He typifies the four-year-old described by the Gesell Institute. And Joy is the typical eighteen-monther. She had two long tantrums this morning.
>
> July 15—This was a day when I felt ready to batter each of the kids. Anne got into my lipstick—Joy had tantrums—Anne and Peter refused to take naps. Peter asked permission to visit a friend, and I gave in; but he had a tantrum when I called him home for supper. Daddy arrived just then and attempted a conversation

with Peter about control. Then Daddy lost control and spanked Peter. But apparently Peter got some idea of the concept, becuase he spoke of control later and said, "Anne, can you say control? Try to say control." After the confrontation with Daddy was over, Peter sat in my lap for about ten minutes. Suddenly he said, "I have enough cuddle now." He left my lap and ate supper peacefully.

Four is sometimes a difficult age for the person who is four as well as for his parents, nursery school teachers and pediatricians. The attitudinal differences of three- and four-year-olds is very clear in the pediatrician's office. Nurses and physicians can approach a three-year-old easily with happy results, but the four-year-old must be handled with extra sensitivity.

Fours can be whiney, irritable, weepy and frequently seem unhappy. They like the phrase, "But I want it" or "I want to do it" or "I don't *want* to do it." They strive for greater independence and self-sufficiency, but they are also insecure. They may resist suggestions or nudges by adults. They seem to enjoy complaining about clothes or food or people. "I don't like that kind." "It's yucky food." "I want to wear something else."

They can lie blatantly and fabricate complicated stories. They may seem devious and untrustworthy to their parents. They are also very creative and have vivid imaginations.

"Did you wash your hands?"

"Yes." (The hands are filthy.)

"Did you take that last cookie?"

"No." (Cookie crumbs on his fingers and cheeks.)

"I went to a castle this morning and played. I was the queen. They gave me jewelry when I was there."

"May I see the jewelry?"

"Somebody took it from me."

Parents, nursery school staff, nurses, physicians can only be understanding and patient. After all, if they follow the book, the "difficult fours" become "angelic fives."

Spanking

We were probably better parents, at least in our theoretical world of child care, before we had any kids. It was easy then to make decisions like "never spank," "never give candy," or "set limits and they'll understand." In that theoretical world the reference to spanking in the previous diary segment could not have occurred. We were convinced that spanking was bad, and we managed to live by that conviction until Peter was about two-and-a-half.

We first broke with the theory over Peter's urges to go running into the street in front of our house. When all the other techniques had failed and after several frightening episodes, I spanked him. He stopped making those wild dashes toward danger.

We have spanked each of our children. Usually it was to stop dangerous behavior. Sometimes it was when we became angry over persistent negative behavior—an hour of screaming by a five-year-old when guests were present or repeated crayoning on the wall by a six-year-old.

A more effective technique in our house was "losing privileges" when, for example, wet pants were discovered hidden for the sixth time, or a child persisted in coming home late from the neighbors'. We tried to be careful in how we worded those consequences. "You lose the privilege; not for wetting, but for hiding the wet pants." And we tried to be alert to reward the child later when he came to whisper, "My wet pants are in the laundry tub."

Am I now rationalizing our use of spanking? Maybe. Some recent research by Dr. Chamberlain at the University of Rochester indicates that friendly, outgoing behavior in children was associated with positive parental contact, such as playing with the child, reading a story, hugging, praising, etc.; but that the specific discipline techniques used were not related to the parents' use of positive contact. Dr. Chamberlain states, "The lack of relationship with parental use of negative contact suggests that the controversy over whether or not to spank is probably irrelevant to the future development of the child."

Obviously, if spanking progresses to beating, battering and child abuse, it can affect the future development of the child. Physicians see infants who are beaten, shaken and burned by their parents. Logic would seem to indicate that children should not be spanked or otherwise punished unless they are of an age and intelligence when they can be told why. But frustrated and angry parents may not be so logical. Some experts see a silver lining in brief outbursts of anger, in that they help clear the air of our pent up frustrations so that positive contact can resume.

Relapsed Toilet Training

Once a child has outgrown a behavior pattern, parents hate to see a relapse, especially if it involves for the parents a return to cleaning soiled underwear. Here's Peter at three-and-a-half:

> July 26—Yesterday Peter had a b.m. in his pants at school. I noted that he came home without underpants and asked why. He replied, "I didn't poop in my pants." Later one of the school attendants dropped off the

rinsed underwear. I made no mention to Peter that she had confirmed that he had had an accident at school.

Tonight he had a bowel movement in the bathtub—in my bathtub as a matter of fact. I had left him in the tub and heard loud yelling, "I want to come out."

When I came into the bathroom he said over and over, "I'm scared, I'm scared," and then I saw the stool in the tub.

I did not scold. Instead I said, "Well, you can't use this tub any more tonight."

I rebathed him and he went to bed without fuss.

When a child who has seemed well toilet trained has relapses in the form of wet or messy pants, we wonder why. Well-read parents tend to look for psychological significance and, indeed, there may be some. The child may be seeking attention. He may be regressing. Or he may have a urinary tract infection or a gastro-intestinal upset. Or he may simply have been busy and forgotten to use the bathroom. In any event, the best attitude is "Wait and see." If the symptoms persist in spite of laissez-faire parental attitudes, the parents are justified in looking for causes.

Nap Time

The need for pre-schoolers to take naps varies with the child and with the tolerance of the parents. Cranky kids in the late afternoon can be perceived as more of a problem by some parents than by others. The need for naps may vary with the number of pre-schoolers in the household. A nap may not be needed if the pre-schooler is an only child or has siblings who are much older, and if neighbor children are not around to stimulate the child to hyperactivity. In settings such as nursery schools in which children are constantly stimulated to heightened activity by one another, it is customary to have a quiet period in the afternoon. Some nursery schools have a resting mat for each child and arrange thirty to sixty minutes of quiet time. In households which have older siblings who encourage the small child to stay up late or awaken him early in the morning, naps may also be more necessary.

In our family we felt that our children needed naps. They did not always perceive it that way. How can parents teach themselves not to project their feelings of fatigue or hunger or cold onto their children? I don't know, and I certainly did a lot of projecting of my own feelings on the day of this diary entry:

> August 13—Last night I went to bed at 4:30 a.m. after delivering a friend's baby. I spent all morning at well-baby clinics and was looking forward to a nice rest with the children. (Joy was nineteen months, Anne was two years, and Peter was three-and-a-half.) Alas, the sequence went like this:
>
> 12:15 I lay down with Anne and Joy in their room. They moved constantly.
>
> 12:30 Peter came home from nursery school, removed his clothes and excited Anne and Joy by talking and laughing.
>
> 12:34 Anne got up to void.
>
> 12:40 Joy got up, same reason.
>
> 12:45 Anne had a bowel movement and tried to clean herself. I cleaned her and then cleaned Peter who was in my bathroom.
>
> 12:50 Peter asked me to sleep with him. Just as I was dozing off I heard loud laughing and talking from

Anne and Joy. Peter began calling to them, then he started fiddling with a key in the closet door. Somehow he hurt his finger and had to have me kiss it.

1:10 Joy got out of bed again. I returned to the girls' room. Joy kept twisting and turning. Anne kicked me.

1:30 Anne and Joy were out of bed again and running around madly.

2:00 I was dead tired. Just as I was dropping into sleep, Peter came pounding on my door.

2:30 Anne and Joy running around. I found them dipping their hands in the toilet bowl and washing their faces. I washed their hands and faces, and returned them to bed. They were subdued for five minutes.

2:35 Our babysitter arrived and I went to sleep immediately.

My problem in this situation was obviously that I was more interested in my own sleep than in theirs and too fatigued to do the soothing which I normally did at nap times. The three children usually slept about an hour in the early afternoon and awakened refreshed and pleasant. If they missed their naps, we were aware of unusual crankiness and hyperactivity in late afternoon and around suppertime.

If a child does not actually go to sleep at nap time, the period can be designated as "quiet time" during which he can sit on his bed and look at books or engage in a quiet game. I have found that the quiet time often evolves into a sleep even for some five-year-olds.

We found it important to keep a regular routine of naps and quiet times. And we found it best if regular naps, regular mealtimes and regular bedtimes could be maintained, if at all possible, during vacations and family moves. This made it easier for the children to adjust to new places: "The scene and the house have changed, but I still have my quiet time after lunch with my own pillow and blanket and favorite toy."

Fears

Parents have fears, some of them rational and others irrational; so do children. Sometimes they may be influenced by the fears of their parents as well as by those of their siblings, playmates and television characters. Some fears, especially those occurring between one and three years, may be part of a child's separation anxiety. Some bedtime difficulties may be based on this, although the mere fear of separation from parents cannot explain all the dilly-dallying that goes on at bedtime.

Some fears in kids are based on genuinely terrifying experiences, such as a fire, a tornado or a dog bite. Some fears are based on a general fear of the unknown. Children vary in this regard, and some with greater fear are more hesitant to explore the unknown.

When Anne was two and Peter was three-and-a-half, we had not yet had a dog in our home. The children had a fear of this unknown.

> August 21—Tonight Anne played her going-away game. Ordinarily she takes my purse, goes down the hall, and returns shortly. Tonight she hid by wrapping herself into about six turns of the living room drapes. I played her game.
>
> "Peter, Anne has gone to the beach. I bet she's having fun. She's playing in the sand and swimming."

Fears

> Anne giggled delightedly, enmeshed in the folds of the curtain. Then the devil prompted me.
>
> "I wonder if she's seeing any dogs on the beach?"
>
> Swiftly the curtains unfurled. Peter and I laughed as the traveler returned in panic, and she also laughed when she saw us.
>
> The children still fear dogs. In fact, two nights ago Peter came into our bed briefly; but he didn't stay, because he imagined that my slippers lying on the floor were dogs.
>
> Two nights ago, Daddy was awakened at 3 a.m. by something scratching his arm. It was Joy, who had been busy writing on his arm and sheet with a ballpoint pen. Her nightly crying and wandering, triggered by her eczema, are fatiguing us. Tonight, in near desperation, I gave her a little Benadryl and will see if that helps.

Fears may be manifested openly or verbally or indirectly. Kids may cry, scream, cling and run. Or they may turn silent and pale, hide themselves, refuse to eat or refuse to play. Sometimes parents can identify the fear and understand its origin; for example, the fear of a doctor's office after having undergone an ear-lancing.

Sometimes an identification of the fear does not lead to an understanding of it. For example, a child may fear riding in a car or fear water.

Some fears can be neither identified nor understood.

Parents should try to undo the fears they can identify. Our children overcame their fear of dogs after we got a puppy. We should reassure our children when they seem to be afraid, even when the fear is incomprehensible to them and to us. We should realize that some of the behavior we class as naughty or attention-seeking may be due to fears.

Fears

Many of the questions asked by children may be related to their fears; for example, questions about death, dark, thunder, hospitals. If we answer these carefully we may be able to diminish their fears.

When Anne says to me, "There are monsters behind that fence, Janey told me," I know that she is really frightened. I must take her by the hand and confirm their non-existence.

About six months later in the diary when Peter was four, we traveled with him to another city for eye surgery. What we did not know at that time was that a six-year-old friend of his had told Peter, "When you get there, those doctors are going to cut your eyes out."

When we arrived, my son seemed very anxious. The first doctor we met was the director of the Children's Hospital and an old friend. When Peter was introduced he promptly kicked the good doctor in the shins and then ran across the room. I was embarrassed. When he learned the surgery was postponed he seemed relieved. But he became tense and morose again later when we tried to explain the coming eye surgery. I couldn't understand this, for I could not recall any bad medical experiences that Peter had had. On the day before surgery he suddenly said, "I won't be having any more birthdays—ever." At that point I was beginning to share his fear. He sensed that, too, for young children tune in to their parents' conscious or unconscious fears.

When the day came he was most cooperative. After the surgery the first thing he said to me was, "I can see. They didn't cut my eyes out."

I asked what he meant, and then I began to comprehend his unexplained fear of the doctors and the surgery. For two months he had lived with a tormenting and unnecessary fear because of a teasing statement by a good friend. Many children have similar prolonged fears because of thoughtless statements made by siblings, friends and adults.

Possessiveness and Sibling Rivalry

It is necessary to a child's emotional well-being that he comprehend the word "me" in relation to himself. He must know that he is an individual, a special person who is separate from all other people. Closely aligned with "me" is "mine," and, by age two, many kids can clutch fiercely at an object and declare it "MINE." Sharing does not seem to be instinctive, but possessiveness develops early in our culture. In this diary segment, our Joy was twenty months, Anne was two, and Peter was going on four.

> September 21—Yesterday Daddy came home with a large red toy Volkswagen which the children could sit in and pedal. It was our bonus for buying our new VW bug. The initial struggle over the little red car was dreadful. Joy, when she had to leave the scene of the struggle for her nap, cried for thirty minutes, even though Daddy very thoughfully put the car in bed with her. Before going to sleep she managed to hurl it across the room. Today Joy has lost all interest in it. She can't pedal anyway. But the struggle goes on between Peter and Anne. I am trying out the concept of "turns," which Peter comprehends, but Anne does not.

It is often discouraging to parents when they note their children and playmates squabbling so much over their possessions. Some children do appear to be naturally more generous than others, but it is rare to see much giving or sharing before age five or six. We tried to teach our children that if a child has strong feelings about objects that belong to him he should also have strong feelings and respect for objects that belong to others. Respect for property rights is basic in our culture, and children can learn this early.

In some cultures it is considered wrong to deny a toddler

anything he wants. Adults and older children must acquiesce to every whim of the youngest, who leads a charmed life until he is no longer a baby. Then comes the rude awakening. A variation of this occurs sometimes in American culture when another child is born after a gap of many years.

Parents and siblings, as role models, can encourage their own values in younger children by demonstrating their belief with respect to sharing, to property rights, and to the importance or insignificance of material possessions. We hope, even while the children squabble about their early possessions, that they will grow up sharing and generous. How happy we were when Joy, on her eighth birthday, heard about another girl from Asia spending her eighth birthday on the very same day in the hospital with no party in sight: Joy split her gifts and spent three hours at the girl's bedside, and they celebrated their mutual birthday together.

Dressing

Children usually begin to take off their clothes by themselves around eighteen months and to put on clothing by two-and-a-half years. The ability to dress oneself is a special developmental milestone and gives a child the sense of pride and independence. Along with the ability to dress come difficulties.

> October 3—(Anne is twenty-seven months) I discovered Anne was dressed in an undershirt, two pairs of panties, one blouse and one pair of shortalls. She insisted she also wanted to wear diapers. I obliged her, and then she wanted pajamas over everything else. I suggested that she put them on herself if she liked, and she did. She continues to have very definite ideas about what she wants to wear and is, of course, totally oblivious to fashion and appropriate dress.

Dressing

Parents, when faced with the sight of summer clothing in winter or best dress for rough play, will discourage self-dressing. The best solution is to limit choices. Put best outfits in another closet. Keep only reasonably appropriate clothing in sight of a child, and then he can dress himself in his choice. It is ironic that a society which can afford more than one change of clothing for its average citizens, including children, has thereby created dressing difficulties not only for toddlers but for teen-agers. The ease with which clothing can be washed, even if it's done by hand, compounds the difficulties. Many changes of clothing are available and if mittens, jackets, shoes get lost, there always seem to be replacements. When my husband went through the lost and found of our local grade school recently, it took him a half hour—boxes and boxes of clothing lost and not reclaimed. Perhaps fewer clothes would help.

Some children may choose not to dress themselves because they enjoy the extra attention they receive while being dressed. It helps to give these children extra praise and attention when they do dress themselves. As children learn to dress themselves, it's obviously a good idea to teach them to put dirty clothes in the hamper or down the chute and to hang up coats, sweaters and dresses. Unfortunately, I don't know how to make the teaching stick. Role-modeling of parents is obviously important in this area. If one or both parents drop their belongings anywhere and everywhere, the offspring are likely to do the same. If one parent is neat and the other messy, the children take the path of least resistance—and, at least in my experience, it turns out to be the messiest!

Reality Concepts

We live in a complicated world where concepts of reality are often hard for an adult to fathom. Yet it is so easy to assume that our children share our adult views of reality. In fact, they are involved in a very elaborate process of fitting themselves and their world into an understandable framework. French psychologist Piaget wrote scholarly volumes on this subject after spending several years observing his own children develop.

Peter was almost four, Anne was three and Joy was two-and-a-half when they were confronted with the reality of daddy on the TV screen.

> November 23—Daddy was on television two nights ago. After the kids had their baths and were in pajamas, we sat in front of the TV to watch the live show. When he appeared on the screen the children became so excited that they seemed hysterical. Joy kept yelling, "Daddy, Daddy." Peter tried to talk with his father on the screen. Anne laughed and laughed and kept looking around the back of the set for Daddy. But after he had been on for five minutes, they became bored and left the TV for other pursuits. Even their own father could not glue them to the TV, which we seldom watch except on such occasions. Nor do the children ask for it.

We smile at two- and three-year-olds who look for daddy behind the televison set because daddy must be inside. But most of their mistaken conceptualizations go unrecognized by us.

The lives of families who live in remote villages are easier for their children to comprehend. Parents do not disappear suddenly or go to mysterious "work." The work is done in the village area. Voices come from relatives and friends, not from telephones and radios. Grandparents, aunts, uncles and cousins are within walking distance and do not materialize out of airplanes arriving from mysterious places. Stool is not flushed down a frightening commode to disappear forever, but is deposited on the ground where children can see it.

Modern children must understand much more complicated environments. As parents we should be on the lookout for misconceptions which might hinder our children's development and happiness.

Early Signs of Creativity

All children are endowed with creative abilities. In varying degrees they may submerge some of these abilities as they mature.

> December 7—This evening we called Peter for his bath, and he didn't answer. I went downstairs, and all was quiet. He was sitting in an overstuffed chair quietly drawing. Perhaps he was so engrossed, at the age of four, that he hadn't heard. The pictures were of cars, which he said were for Grandma. He was also writing his name "EPTER."
>
> After baths I was intrigued to find Daddy lying on the bed in the girls' room doing a countdown for Peter and Anne, who were on their way to the moon. "We are playing spaceship," said Peter.
>
> They were dressed in spacesuits—Plastic pants over slacks, coats, hats—and they were putting items representing food, water, etc., in their "spaceship," which was the wardrobe closet. Finally they scrunched themselves in. Daddy counted down; and, whoosh, they were off. After a few seconds they reached the moon, climbed out of their spaceship and walked on the moon.

I pointed to Anne. "There's pretty moon-girl."

She giggled and pointed to Peter. "See, there moon-boy."

We never played such games when we were kids.

Joy did not join the spaceship game, but spent the time hugging and kissing Mama and Daddy. She is very affectionate now.

Creativity is difficult to define. We can easily recognize this quality in a Beethoven symphony or a Renoir painting; but it is harder to recognize that creative individuals are those who can occupy themselves without aid of other humans or materials, who can make a hovel appear beautiful, who can entertain others and who are never bored. Children are endowed with vivid imaginations, and this is exemplified in their imaginary games and friends and stories. And how sad to see some children at four and five who are already too concrete to join in the wonderful games of imagination.

Creativity in children enables them to turn knickknacks into golden serving dishes and mud into magnificent collages. It enables them to take on new roles. It enables them to sit for hours with pencil and paper as they transmit imagery to paper. It enables them to tell stories, compose poems, compose songs. Creativitiy keeps them frightfully busy and messy and happy. Our concrete, dull, compulsive parental selves must restrain the impulses to squelch their creative activities, lest they grow up bored and uncreative.

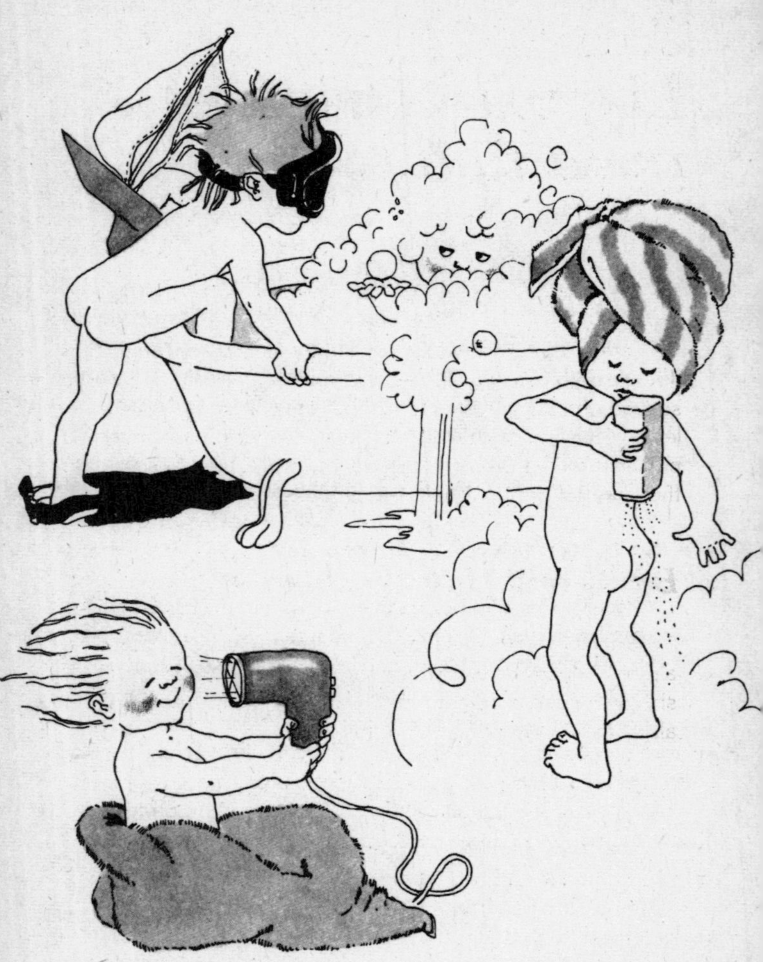

Although children can assist in their own bathing and shampooing while they are still pre-schoolers, they require supervision.

3
Life with children aged two to five

Peter had now turned four, Anne was two-and-a-half, and Joy was almost two. It was the year of a family move, the second one in two years for us, but the children survived it at least as well as their parents. I was working part-time as a pediatrician both before and after the move, but I was still with the children during most of their waking hours.

Baths and Hair Washing

Since we Americans tend to bathe our kids and ourselves almost beyond the tolerance of normal skin, the least we should require is that our bathing not be a grim necessity, but also fun for the kids and the parents.

> January 2—We spent New Year's Day with the neighbors, and our kids had a wonderful, active time with their two-year-old and infant. They were falling asleep in the car en route home. We skipped the usual bedtime baths and tucked them in immediately when we reached home around 7 p.m. It seems to me that the before-bedtime bathing ritual is very pleasant for the kids and for me, and it's a necessity as well because of the ubiquitous red clay around our yard.

Baths and Hair Washing

> January 4—Anne is obsessed with water these days and runs to the sink whenever we aren't watching to fill whatever she can with water. She gives drinks to her dollies and to herself and washes toys and dollies frequently. She also resists coming out of the tub. Tonight the little imp threw Peter's wooden puzzle into his bath—which he enjoyed, but I didn't.

Traditionally bathing has been both a cleansing and a soothing ritual. A warm bath or shower can be a relaxing beginning or ending to a day, and children often regard it as such. Fancy commercial bath toys are available, but children will enjoy empty plastic bottles, plastic food containers, jar caps, cans, or small rubber dolls as well. If baths become a reason for resistance, parents may decrease their frequency for awhile. Children often like to wash themselves, but it is important not to stress the scrubbing aspect of the bath. In particular, the vaginal area of little girls should not be scrubbed. This can denude the thin epithelial covering and cause chapping irritation and even infection of the perineum. Likewise, care should be taken that children do not use excessive soap or forget the soap bar at the bottom of the tub. If children have dry skin, soaps should be used as little as possible, and preferably only superfatted varieties should be used. Bubble baths can cause bladder irritation, especially in girls, and are best avoided. Showers are preferable to baths if dry skin is a problem and, to prevent drying, a non-perfumed cream can be rubbed on after bathing when the skin is still slightly moist.

Hair washing can be a happy time if the shampooer is careful to avoid soap in the eyes. Many children enjoy having their hair shaped into "rabbit ears," "squirrel ears," or "topknots" while the soap is in. They then observe themselves in the mirror with great hilarity. Although children can assist in their own bathing and shampooing while they are still pre-schoolers, they require supervision. We have felt that they should not be left to bathe themselves until they are school age, and we have controlled the bath temperature selection until age eight or nine.

Pica

Pica is a medical term for the eating or chewing of items that are not food. A certain amount of pica is normal in the infant and toddler periods. Part of early exploration is learning how things taste.

Even though I have no recollection of eating dirt in my life, I think I know exactly how it tastes; and I suspect that most adults recollect that taste just as well as I. Perhaps what we recall are early memories of the surreptitious tastes we took when we were toddlers.

But now that we are parents, pica is understandably one of the things that can worry us about our children, as it did the day of the birthday party at the Reilleys':

> January 25—The children and their parents had a wonderful time. The kids brought home coloring books, crayons, balloons, candy and paper hats. I put them to bed at 7:30, but they weren't ready to sleep. While Daddy and I were eating, we heard a lot of commotion upstairs. I went up and found Joy with a big wad of orange paper hat in her mouth and a very orange tongue. I washed her mouth with water several times. Now I am wondering what poisons may have been in the paper.

> January 26—Today Joy's urine was orange-colored. And as if that weren't bad enough, I saw a piece of balloon in her stool. When I picked her up from the

> Sunday school nursery, she had yellow crayon chewed up inside her mouth. I told Daddy I thought we should give her a pipe to chew on constantly—just like Daddy.

Joy seemed to have the greatest sucking requirement of the children. We attributed this to the lonely months she had experienced in an orphanage. However, there seem to be some children whose fondness for sucking things is apparent at birth, before one could interpret it as a substitute for lack of attention. Some infants suck in utero.

Some researchers have tried to associate pica with various deficiency states such as iron deficiency. This has not been proved. Because pica can cause physical harm, we worry more about it than habits such as sucking a thumb or blanket or pacifier. If a child swallows paper and buttons and pennies and matchsticks, the result might be intestinal obstruction or perforation. If she chews and swallows paint chips or plaster containing lead, she may become poisoned by the lead. She might choke on some things. And from dirty objects she could develop intestinal infections.

Remonstrations and punishment are unlikely to cure pica even in children of school age. Young children need watching, and I obviously didn't watch closely enough on the afternoon of the birthday party. It has been suggested that snack foods which require a lot of chewing may help to reduce the risk from pica. Sugarless chewing gum may fall in this category, but I do not recommend gum for children under age four. Fortunately, as chidlren grow older they tend to use more discretion in what they chew.

Neighbor Children

When Anne was two-and-a-half we recorded these entries about her early lessons in socialization in the neighborhood.

They involved a big boy, Philip, almost six years old, who lived across the street.

> February 1—I was amused last night to note that little mother Anne was sleeping on the very edge of her single bed, but that the bear she had inherited from Philip was very comfortably lying square in the middle of her pillow, well covered with all the blankets. She was sleeping very uncomfortably in order to insure comfort for her baby.
>
> February 7—Daddy has decided that the bear represents Philip to Anne, and I think he is right. I hadn't realized how much she wants Philip's approval and attention for everything she does, until I observed a supper here when Philip stood by. "Look, Philip, I am eating my food first." "Philip, do you want some of my meat?" "Philip, come and sit by me." Philip is the big brother here—no doubt about that. Interesting how they all play together day-after-day-after-day without serious altercations.

Children can learn much about socialization within their neighborhoods. When our children were pre-schoolers we preferred to have the neighbor children at our home rather than vice versa. So neighbor children were often around, and we felt it was important to maintain a positive attitude toward them. Neighbor children, like our own, could be interesting, nice, mean, threatening, charismatic, frightening, enjoyable, bothersome, helpful, dominating, rude—and sometimes a single child could manifest many of these characteristics in one day.

Sometimes older children take out feelings of hostility and aggression on smaller children, and sometimes little children follow older children into activities beyond their capacity.

Thus, as parents, we should expect to follow the course of activities involving our children and neighbors. My own efforts in this regard have been far from perfect. Sometimes a phone call was all the distraction needed to keep me from watching at crucial times. Our catalog of disasters included a black eye suffered by Peter when a bigger girl decided to beat him with a stick, and a bad scare when an unhappy older child dumped a pail of sand over Joy's head and eyes. There was also an arm laceration that occurred when Peter tried to intervene in a dog fight.

If we observe hostile, aggressive or cruel behavior in our own or the neighbor children who are playing together, we separate them for a period of several days. And we expect that they will do better next time.

Moving with Young Children

When Peter was four, Anne was going on three, and Joy two, we moved our family to a new home in a new city.

> April 5—We are moving in four days. Today the neighbors had a farewell lunch for us. The children ate at a table by themselves and did very well. The children are busy messing in all the objects we bring out to pack. Tonight Joy took (or didn't take) a lick of Renuzit which I had in a pile of things to leave with the neighbors. Peter doesn't want to comprehend that we are leaving permanently. I haven't emphasized this aspect of our forthcoming trip to a new home. He talks of coming back.

> April 11—We left by air on a rainy morning and the kids seemed to take the departure calmly. The plane

trip was long; but there were extra seats for our family, and they were able to play and sleep in comfort.

April 16—Peter has seemed to be regressing these past three days with some crying and kicking episodes, and Joy has had frequent tantrums. I tell myself to forget the cleaning and arranging and try to spend much time playing with them, reading, going for walks outside.

April 26—Daddy took the kids out for a couple of rides today. He also showed them movies of themselves in our former home. They were just thrilled—even Joy. "Hi," they said to their friends. "Those people in our walls," Anne called them.

May 9—Tonight I continued with the stories about Leslie, Stevie and Boo-Boo—stories I have made up about a five-year-old boy, his four-year-old sister and two-and-a-half-year-old Boo-Boo. The children were terribly rapt and interested. Leslie, Stevie and Boo-Boo have gone through a move from one house to another; Boo-Boo gets lost. Our kids beg me to repeat over and over what they call the "Boo-Boo Song."

The average American family moves once every five years; therefore, the average child will probably be part of at least one move before he or she reaches school age. Young children form attachments to their homes, to neighbors, to babysitters; and they might be confused or upset by the sudden disappearance of what is loved and familiar. Moving can also be a growing, enriching, positive experience for parents and children; although many parents, teachers, pediatricians and psychiatrists feel that there is a point when moves become too frequent and contribute to insecurity and unhappiness in children. When moves must be made, the following efforts may help pre-schoolers to understand, accept, and possibly even enjoy them:

1. Tell the children stories about moving. Explain the positive aspects of the move to them. Try to verbalize their concerns about moving.

2. Allow children to select a few treasured toys, blankets or other objects to accompany them directly during their move.

3. Avoid leaving toys, children's books, bicycles, etc., in storage, for these then become lost to the kids and only increase their insecurities.

4. Avoid prolonged transitional periods in neighbors' houses, hotels, motels, temporary housing.

5. At least initially, attempt to duplicate the child's previous sleeping arrangement as much as possible with the same bed, blankets, pictures, toys, etc., in the sleeping room.

6. Parents, or at least one parent, should plan to stay home nights with children during first weeks in a new home. A new home, new environment, and new babysitter all at once are unsettling to young children.

7. Take time for activities which the children enjoy during first weeks in a new place. Take care that the children do not feel displaced by parents' preoccupations with new friends, unpacking, new jobs, licenses, or shopping.

Children are unlikely to fear air travel, but it is still a good idea to discuss a planned first flight in detail with them. We emphasized the positive aspects—the thrill of being in the sky, the speed, the soft drinks and the meals—but we also told them that seat belts were required and running in aisles was not allowed.

If children are under six, a long flight should be arranged with regard to their sleeping hours. Flights during the night or during nap time make life much easier for parents. I do not usually recommend sedatives for children, but a sedative in reserve can be useful during a flight with young children. Children who get airsick can be given an anti-emetic before a flight. Children should not fly when they have colds or other contagious illnesses. Diarrhea on a flight can be a nuisance to parents and an annoyance to other passengers.

Those Terrible Twos

The very phrase "terrible twos" is bad programming. The behavior of persons in their second and third years of life probably lends itself to more categorizing and predicting than that of any other years. Two-year-olds are playful, fun-loving, energetic, easily influenced by role models, and also exasperating at times. How tolerant I could be of someone else's two-year-old, but how angry I could become over the tantrums of my own!

Here's our Joy at twenty-seven months:

April 30—Joy has been yelling angrily and crying for forty-five minutes as I record this at 11 p.m. I put her to bed at 9:00. She began crying and said that she wanted to sleep with Peter. When Peter agreed, she lay quietly with him for two minutes and then said she wanted her crib. I put her back—relative quiet for thirty minutes—and then she began yelling, "I need a sheet. I need diapers." I investigated; found her lying in the nude. I replaced her clothes, messaged her itching skin with cream, and put her to bed. There was immediate crying again. After ten minutes I returned once more, gave her water, replaced the blanket, and patted her back for a few minutes. Then I said, "Good night, Joy. I'm going to bed."

I went to bed. Then came, "Scratch me, Mommy, scratch me." Her voice becoming more and more angry as I didn't respond. This for five minutes.

"I need blankie—I need blankie—RIGHT NOW." She kept this up for ten minutes intermingled with enraged crying.

"I baby, Mama, I baby, Mama." (Trying to coax me back.)

Occasionally she yelled, "Daddy, Daddy." (He wasn't home.)

"I need to go wee-wee. I need to go wee-wee." (Five minutes.)

"I want a drink. I want a drink." (I became fascinated by her persistence.)

"I am hurting—need medicine." (Ten minutes of this gimmick.)

"I am very tired, Mommy. I am very tired, Mommy."

When she began the series anew I began writing; and while I was writing, she got out of the crib and stood at my door saying, "I want to say goodnight to Anne" for five minutes. When she finally opened my door I got up without a word and looked at her sternly. Immediately she said quickly, "I want to say goodnight to Anne." I led her to Anne who was sleeping. Then Joy said, "Now I want to say goodnight to Peter." I led her to him. She lay down by him. Then, "Blankie, blankie. I want blankie." Again this went on for five minutes.

Now she is outside my door again. "I want my pillow. I want to sleep with you. Mommy, where are you?

Hurting, Mommy. Where is Daddy, Mommy?" At times her tone was conversational and at times angry.

There she stands, and it is after 11. What am I to do?

I took her back to her crib, returned to my bed and tried to relax. She came back to my door, yelled something about Anne, then slowly opened the door.

"I want to say goodnight to you, Mommy. I good girl. My blankie is over there. I want it." She said this several times and edged to the mattress, grabbed her blanket and went out, leaving my door open. I made no response.

A few minutes later she said twice, "Mommy, close your door." Still no response from me. At 11:30 she returned, shut my door, and all was quiet. At 11:45 I investigated. She had also shut the children's door and was sound asleep in Peter's bed. I had not said a word to her for one-and-a-half hours. I had ignored her, but she surely did not ignore me.

Two-year-olds are often ambivalent. They want independence, but they need their parents. They manifest their self will by negativism and tantrums. When this is combined with their need to explore at this age, the results are sometimes exasperating. And no method works with every two-year-old. The old adage, "Ignore their outbursts," sometimes works and sometimes doesn't. It definitely doesn't work if they refuse to be ignored. It's probably a good idea to avoid giving them secondary gain* from their tantrums. On the other hand, if their tantrum occurs in a supermarket or department store, it's a little hard to ignore them.

*Secondary gain means attention or other fringe benefit derived from an action.

For us the best solution was to think of the future when they would be three or four or five, more certain of their independence and less prone to tantrums. And now when I reread the diary and remember the charm of my once two-year-olds, I miss them!

Blaming

Children learn early to blame others for their failings and misdeeds. Anne was not yet three when we recorded this entry:

> June 24—At bedtime I have been telling the kids stories of when they were babies. They like this very much. Sometimes we review details of days—"What we did today," "What we did yesterday," or "Peter's day at the hospital." They love it.
>
> This morning we awakened to find Anne and Peter in bed with us. There was a wet spot on my side where Anne had been lying. I asked, "Who wet my bed?" Promptly Anne said, "Joy did."
> "But she's not even here," I said.
> Anne stoutly insisted that Joy had been the culprit.

The tendency to blame others whenever possible is learned from early role models, and that presumably includes parents. In spite of our better intentions we at times blame them when it serves no useful end to do so. They counter by blaming others. Obviously we should discourage the blaming reaction.

Yet we need to teach our children responsibility for their actions, and we should help them to make the necessary amends for their actions. A six-year-old who scratches his name on someone else's bedroom door should be told that it is his responsibility to remove the scratches. As parents, we can show him how to use sandpaper and how to restain the wood; but ideally the child should do the work and receive a minimum of secondary gain in the process. Then we can say: "You scratched the door, but you also fixed it. That's great. The bad mistakes are the ones that are much harder than that to fix."

If one of our children persists in blaming others, we sometimes use the phrase, "Let me hear you say something nice about her. I don't want to hear about mistakes." Or, "We all make mistakes. Let's think about the good things he does."

Anger and Hostility

Sometimes children get mad—as do parents, and special interest groups and nations. Almost all of us learned, when young, that anger sometimes got results when other reactions did not. Anger became something we expected in ourselves and in others, and sometimes we rationalized that the anger was good. Children learn expressions of anger from role models; and they, in turn, become role models. Thus, at four-and-a-half, one of our children demonstrated that he could verbalize feelings of anger. Peter had invited his five-year-old friend, David, home to spend the night with us.

> July 24—David seemed very happy until his father called. Then he began to cry and insisted on going home. So his parents fetched him. Peter was angry because David left. This morning he said, "I was mad at you, Mama, so I ate the vitamins." Belatedly I realized that last night, after David left, Peter had finished off the chewable vitamins (about ten).

Peter had been frustrated, hurt and angry when his friend left him abruptly. He needed some attention. Perhaps he wanted to express his distress to David or his parents, but they had left. So he took a course many of us take. He transferred his angry feeling to someone else. He chose to do something he knew I would not like. Regrettably he did not tell me immediately, either because he was tired and fell asleep or because he recalled the stomach pumping he had almost experienced at age two.

Children learn quickly in social situations that overt expressions of anger are unacceptable. The transfer of angry feelings has often become a reality in our household. When one of the children comes home from school slamming doors or hitting siblings, we have learned to look for the original trigger for the anger.

If we are able to ask quietly, "What made you angry today?" the child will often explain the problem. Sometimes the anger is directed at oneself because of a failure to perform or receive or be nominated. Sometimes neither the child nor the parent can figure them out, but at least we can agree that the angry feelings are not a reaction to something a member of the household has done to the child.

The models of anger and violence in our society have been pervasive, but mercifully we seem to be reducing them. In the medical and mental health professions there is a strong interest in studying the effects of TV violence on our children. The findings so far point to a compelling need for a new national consensus on the contents of our public entertainment. We can expect such a consensus to develop rapidly once the effects of our constant exposure to the cult of violence are understood and communicated.

Threats and Rewards

Threats from a small child can be both disconcerting and amusing for a parent. By the time our third child, Joy, was two-and-a-half, we had had enough experience with pre-schoolers to be relatively casual about the technique.

> August 19—We've had a pleasant evening with the kids. They've been very happy during the past week, except I've noted that Joy has begun using threats. She says, "I'm going to throw you in the garbage can if you don't give me gum." I remember Peter using the identical threat at the same age, but probably not for the same reason. He didn't know about the wonders of gum because he had no older brother or sister to announce its virtues.

If I had been dumped in the garbage pail as many times as it has been threatened me, I would long since have turned into compost. Some of the threats from pre-schoolers demonstrate original thinking.

"If you don't let me go to Doug's house, I'll throw my shoes away."

"If you won't give me chewing gum, I'll cry all day."

"If you won't buy me a bicycle, I'll kill you."

Children develop the use of threats, albeit ridiculous ones, at a very early age. They learn this technique from their parents.

"Let's pick up the playroom quickly so we can go to visit Aunt Jenny."

"No dessert unless you eat your peas."

"If those coats don't get on in a hurry, we're not going."

"When you have finished brushing your teeth, I'll read you a story."

No matter how sweetly one makes such statements, they still imply threats, and thus initiate our children into the reward system. So we should not be too surprised or angry when children try to coerce us through use of threats of their own. Children realize that they cannot carry out the majority of their fanciful threats and do not expect acquiescence. But sometimes parents do yield, and this might encourage children to use the same techniques later in life.

Few of us like to yield to very demanding or negative-type threats. If the child says, "Give me a penny or I'll scribble on the table," the answer had best be "No." However, if a child says, "Mommy, if I scrub the table and chairs, would you give me a penny?"—depending on the personality of the child and the mood of the mother—she might say, "Yes."

It is important to resolve never to threaten a child with a statement or action which represents a withdrawal of parental love, and not to counter threats from children with threats of our own. The threats of two- and three-year-olds, to some extent, represent their magical thinking and their wish for independence and power. They are best treated with disinterest or gentle rebuttal.

Reaction to Stress

Children, like their parents, react to stress in a variety of ways, reflecting both their innate characteristics and what they have learned about coping. Peter was almost five when we recorded this entry:

> November 1—Peter was going out the front door to take some overripe apples to the pony when he pushed his arm through the storm door window Daddy had installed the previous day. I was in the bathroom with Anne and Joy when it happened. Peter ran to me, and his first words were, "Mama, the door is broken and

> I'm bleeding." Our neighbors helped us with the girls, and we took him to the local emergency room where he had three stitches put into the laceration on his wrist. Fortunately the flying glass had missed his eyes, but he had a few minor scratches around his eyes. Peter cried during preparation for the repair but said only "ouch" during the actual suturing and tetanus booster. Coming home I said, "Peter, I'm sorry you had this bad experience." "It wasn't bad, Mama," he said. "It was fun."

In the shattered door episode Peter seemed to be coping better than his mother. Once again I tried to project my feelings onto him. What we adults think must hurt or be a bad experience need not hurt or be a bad experience. My children have taught me this over and over, and slowly I'm learning. Fortunately, Peter's innate optimism won out over my perception of a "bad experience." Ideally we should all learn to face stress, deal with it appropriately and move on. Children should be allowed to cry if they wish, to verbalize feelings (theirs, not ours) and to recognize the difference between major and minor problems.

Infants face stresses, and there are innate differences in their responses. Some scream for a short time, some scream for a long time, and some withdraw completely. Parents should recognize these innate tendencies when they act as models in a stressful situation.

If a child is very fearful and hides in the face of thunder and lightning, parents should comfort him and do nothing to reinforce the child's fear. If, on the other hand, a child is not fearful of thunder and lightning, parents can explain that it is unwise to go swimming during an electrical storm.

If parents overreact to pain, their children are likely to do the same. If parents moan over lost possessions, dental appointments, a dent in the fender and other minor stresses, their kids may also become overreactors and poor copers. Children are more likely to be calm in the face of major stresses if they sense calmness in their parents. They will learn how to pick up the pieces and move forward instead of regressing in the face of stress.

Of the multitude of skills and abilities a child develops to prepare him for adult life, the ability to cope well with stress is a very useful one to have.

"Stop That, Ocean"

Fortunately for us parents, the frustrations which preschoolers manifest at being thwarted are not directed toward parents only. Here's Joy at twenty-two months.

> November 25—Joy was enjoying herself drawing pictures in the sand today. I observed her as waves crept closer and sloshed over her pictures, taking them away. She glared out toward the ocean, stomped her feet in the sand and yelled over and over, "Stop that, Ocean." It reminded me of the time when Peter, at the same age, had said, "Daddy, turn off the rain."

It takes a lot of ego strength to scold an ocean. As young children realize that they are themselves and separate from all other humans, they yearn for independence and control. It is frustrating to realize that they can't or don't always have such independence or control. One of the positive aspects of a two-year-old's reactions is that they are obvious and unmistakable. As children mature, the same frustrations are manifested less openly and less directly.

Babysitters

In most cultures of the world, parents need look no further than the extended family for babysitters. In our culture our relatives rarely live in the same neighborhood. One parent, usually the mother, can end up with an intolerable amount of being tied to the children. So we need babysitters. They cover for working parents and allow parents an occasional evening out.

> December 7—Last night Daddy and I went out, a rare event for us now. Debby, a teen-age neighbor girl, was our babysitter. Apparently all went well, although the kids don't know her very well.
>
> Mrs. Benke, who watches the children at her house on Thursdays, has made the girls' lamb costumes for the school Christmas play. Yesterday after school, we stopped at Mrs. Benke's to try on the costumes. Joy wanted to keep her costume on and didn't understand that we were trying on a basted article of clothing; thus, she kicked and screamed her way back into the car.

For a working mother like myself, Mrs. Benke fulfilled two priceless attribues of a babysitter: She had a spontaneous love for chldren, and our relationship with her continued over an extended period of time. Debby, too, became a regular and well-liked babysitter in the years ahead. In the above diary segment she represented an unknown and therefore a high-risk babysitting solution.

Between the ages of six and twenty-four months, children find separation from their parents especially difficult. It helps them through this period if they have become accustomed to another caretaker or two from early infancy. Leaving them with strangers at this age should be avoided if at all possible.

Babysitters

Unless the babysitting is to be done for occasional brief periods, it is best to think of a prospective babysitter as someone who will stay with a family for years. If a babysitter is being hired for full-time work, or if day-care is being considered, time spent in careful selection is well spent. When both parents intend to work outside of the home, it is worthwhile to allow days or weeks for orienting the babysitter in the home. Children can become accustomed to the babysitter in the presence of a parent who can later spend work days away from home with more assurance that the babysitter is well oriented and that the children are contented.

In selecting a parent surrogate the most important factor is whether the person enjoys children in general and yours in particular. It is also important, of course, that the babysitter is knowledgeable and experienced and that parents determine whether or not the attitudes about child-rearing methods of the babysitter are compatible with their own. How do the parents feel about the age for toilet training, and how does the babysitter feel? Are their views on television watching compatible? If they will be taking their children to the babysitter's home, what sort of lunch and snacks will be served? If a babysitter wants to spoon feed the child until eighteen or twenty-four months, and the parents prefer that he learn to eat by himself at fifteen months, there will be inconsistency in rearing patterns. If they cannot convince a proposed babysitter of their method, they'd better look for someone else. On the other hand, if a babysitter has handled many children and is a professional in knowing how to relate to small children, parents may learn from her (him) and might do better to cooperate with her (his) methods in such matters as toilet training.

Babysitters are necessary when working parents have infants and toddlers at home. After children reach school age it is usually preferable if working parents can make their working hours coincide with school hours, and so do without a babysitter. A school age child is influenced by teachers, schoolmates and neighbor children, whether or not his parents are working outside the home; and the influence of a babysitter therefore assumes less of importance than in the case of a pre-school child.

Our rule was that parents should *not* leave sick children with a babysitter even when the child seemed to have only a minor cold or fever. We also felt that until children were age five or over we should avoid vacations which would leave children behind, unless they were in the care of a relative who was like a household member to the children. Children feel most insecure and concerned about parental absences at night and should not be subjected to the trauma of awakening with a semi-stranger looking at them.

When we used a babysitter for an evening we found it useful to explain to our children where we were going and to stress that we would be back. We often gave the babysitter some previously hidden game or treat to use in entertaining the children. Some parents tape-record themselves reading a story and ask the sitter to play it back while they are gone, but we never went that far. Children will often prefer certain sitters and request them, and we tried to indulge these preferences when possible.

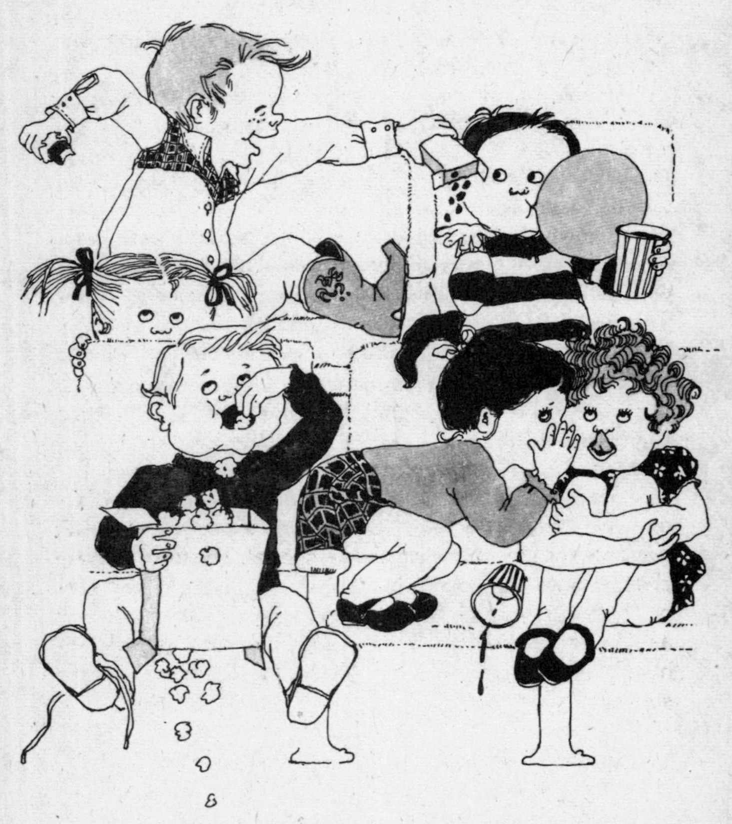

I learned that taking six 4 year olds to the movies is a mistake.

4
Life with children aged three to six

Time was flying. All our babies and toddlers were gone; and in their place, we had three pre-schoolers attending nursery schools part-time while I practiced medicine part-time. The diary year starts with Peter just turned five, Anne at three-and-a-half, and Joy about to celebrate her third birthday.

Birthdays

A home full of kids means you'll have a year full of birthdays. Birthday celebrations are important because they can reinforce the idea that each child is special. The form of these celebrations can depend on many things—number and ages of children, available time and money, traditional customs and the interests of the parents and children. Our celebrations have changed over the years. When Joy was three we were still quite traditional.

> January 9—While the girls were napping I made Joy's birthday cake. She had requested a cherry cake with pink frosting. I left the cake cooling and decided to take a brief nap myself. I fell asleep for a few minutes and awakened to hear some rustling in the living room. I went to find Joy sitting there, her pants wet, poking

holes in an envelope with a pencil. She looked a bit guilty. I found out why when I went to the kitchen. One of the small chairs had been pushed up to the counter, and someone had taken a large chunk from the center of the cake. When I asked Joy if she had done this, I got no response. I didn't press the issue except to say I was sorry she had ruined her own birthday cake. Then I put her in the bathtub, where she was very happy as she pretended to be cooking with her small pots and pans in the tub. Periodically she asked me to taste her cake, then her cookies, chocolate, and other goodies which she was preparing in the tub. About 3 p.m. Daddy came in and took the kids to the basement to play, and I tried to save the cake.

January 10—This was the day Joy had awaited for months—her third birthday. The pink cherry cake looked lovely. We also had carrot cake and open-face sandwiches in the Scandinavian tradition. The children went to church with Daddy while I made last minute preparations—scrubbing the kitchen floor, preparing the tables—two small ones for the the children in the playroom. I even got out the good silver. Guests began arriving before naps were over. These included adults who were special in Joy's life as well as half a dozen children. Joy had a very happy day. The only minor flaw was that she wet her pants in the excitement of play.

We invited significant adults to our birthday parties because that was the tradition in which my husband and I had been raised. When we had lived in areas where relatives were scarce, we usually invited the parents of the children's friends. (These were usually our friends as well. Not surprisingly, current friends of parents with young children tend to be other parents with young children.)

Our early attempts to vary the birthday party routine were not too successful. I learned, for instance, that taking six four-year-olds to the movies is a mistake. But after seventeen innings of serving cake and ice cream plus lawn games and donkey's tails with huge numbers of children, I finally reached the limit of my tolerance for traditional birthday celebrations.

Our current family birthday tradition is an event on or near the birth date of the lucky child, which includes the immediate family and occasionally a cousin or aunt and uncle of the child's choosing. Thus we have had evenings of pizza and roller skating, days of skiing, movies, and banana splits instead of cakes.

In the summer around Children's Day, we have a giant party held outside to which each child may invite five guests. Rain is a chance we take. There are no gifts, but lots of games, picnic food and fun. When our children reach adolescence we predict another change in the form of birthday celebrations.

Reading Readiness

The ability to read is a necessary tool to gain an education in our culture. Its acquisition implies that a child probably has average intelligence, yet there are many gifted persons who do not read well.

Many two- and three-year-olds can be taught reading if someone spends sufficient time teaching them. In fact, many three- and four-year-olds learn letters, reading and writing on their own. The unanswered question is, "Is there a great advantage if one acquires reading skills before four or five or six years?" If reading comes at the expense of other more natural and necessary stages of development, then there may be disadvantages from early reading. If the child learns to read on his own because he wants to, this is probably good. Some young children become seized with learning to write because they wish to write poems, stories and letters. But some of these same children are unable to write very well because they have not acquired the necessary fine motor skills. Vision does not become 20/20 until around six years, and visual ability affects reading and writing skills. Five- and six-year-olds often reverse letters because of perceptual difficulties.

We were ambivalent about teaching our pre-schoolers to read, as illustrated in these two diary excerpts. In the first excerpt, Joy was three and Peter was five. In the second excerpt, Anne was four and Peter was almost six and in kindergarten.

> January 25—Today Joy decided she was no longer Joy. She said that Joy had gone away and that she was Hamy (pronounced Hay-me). She insisted that I was not "Mama," but "teacher," and she would address me as "teacher." I went along with her for a while. I would say, "Hamy, would you like an orange?" She answered, "I'll go ask my mama." She then left the kitchen to chat with her imaginary mother and returned to say, "Yes, she says I can have an orange." By evening Hamy was forgotten.
>
> Peter is asking us to spell words, and he practices writing them. He can read many words without having had any formal training and seems ready to read. In fact he begs to learn to read. However, his nursery school teachers feel that reading should not be stressed at five, and perhaps they are right.
>
> October 29—It was a beautiful afternoon. We worked outside. I did some digging for a tulip bed. Peter was busy with hammer and nails making a table which "You can use for a table at your Halloween party,

> Mama. Won't that be good?" Joy was busy digging in the driveway gravel. Later we made cookies. Peter can read a lot now and sounds out the words he sees on TV. Anne also constantly asks me how to spell words.

We did not practice reading with our children when they were pre-schoolers, although I was tempted to when the kids were asking to learn to read. I don't think that there is a single answer with respect to what is right on this question. Each child is unique, and some are ready to read at earlier ages than others.

Some European school systems have traditionally taught rigorous, structured reading and writing to five-year-olds. Most learning in early years in these school systems was by rote. These children learned to read well, recite well and write beautifully. Examinations at age eleven or twelve decided who was capable of receiving lycee or high school pre-university education. Performance in such exams is dependent on reading ability, and some gifted individuals might miss the opportunity for advanced education because of inadequate reading ability. Rapid readers who comprehend and retain what they read have an advantage in our educational system, but this ability does not necessarily equate with brilliance. In the United States it is possible for persons who lack good reading ability to get college degrees.

To force early reading may be detrimental to normal development in other areas. After all, a three-year-old is a three-year-old and must do certain things before he can be four; but eventually there is pressure on every child to learn to read and write.

Looking back now, we can recall our sighs of relief each time it became apparent that one of our children was learning to read without any major difficulty. When this milestone was passed by our fourth child we were left with nothing more momentous than the math facts to consume the worrier in us. That, too, is passing.

Every problem resolved can breed another if we let it do so, as illustrated by this entry when Peter had just turned seven:

December 27—En route home from my office the children and I stopped at the library. We checked out nine books. Peter has already read his two Christmas Hardy Boys books, read one of the books we got from the library last night, and now has just one remaining. He reads incredibly fast and all the time. There are times when he is so engrossed in a book that he seems totally out of communication. Daddy thinks he should be reading "better literature" than the Hardy Boys.

Concepts of Property and Ownership

Peter was six when I recorded this in the diary:

March 30—Yesterday en route home from school we decided to stop at the neighborhood store for milk and some vegetable seeds. The kids came into the store with me. Ordinarily I don't get out of the car—Peter runs in and buys the milk himself. But yesterday I had to choose the seeds; and while I was looking at seeds, Peter looked at a lovely homemade cake which a lady had left at the store on consignment, hoping for a little cash income. Peter's finger reached out and pushed on the Saran Wrap which covered the cake, and he made a huge indentation in the rich frosting. I said immediately that I would buy the cake. The store manager said, "Never mind, the cake has been here for two days." I

> insisted we pay for it, but he would take only two dollars. On the way home I talked about articles in stores belonging to the store owners and how unfortunate it was that Peter had ruined a cake belonging to someone else. Peter was glum. When we arrived home he ran to his camera bank, which contains about five dollars. He took out two dollar bills and silently handed them to me. I accepted them. All was well.

On vacation later the same year, Anne joined Daddy and me while we were visiting a friend in a neighboring apartment. Anne was four-and-a-half.

> December 31—She seemed to be content to sit quietly on my lap for fifteen minutes; then she left the apartment. Susan, the babysitter, returned with both girls after a few minutes and handed me a little box containing thirteen pieces of bubble gum. I took the gum, which Susan said Anne had bought, and returned it to the little store where they confirmed that Anne had, indeed, been the purchaser.
>
> "Where did you get the money?" I asked.
>
> Repeatedly Anne said, "I'm sorry, but I forgot. I'm sorry, but I forgot."
>
> I persisted "Did you take it?"
>
> "Yes."
>
> "From where?"
>
> "From that man's apartment."
>
> She had taken a quarter from a table in the apartment we were visiting and bought twenty-five pieces of bubble gum. She and friends had consumed twelve within a few minutes. Daddy gave her a quarter and accompanied Anne back to Mr. Daniel's apartment. Shortly after they returned she went to her bed and

sobbed for twenty minutes. Later she came to me and said, "Don't talk about what I did. I can't stand to hear about it. And I won't do it again." I have a feeling that she won't.

Stealing is perhaps too strong a word for acts of pre-school children. They have a limited comprehension of property rights and ownership, and their intent in taking something is not to deprive someone else. Yet, when caught, they will act guilty. They will fabricate stories (four-year-olds are especially adept at this) to explain how someone else's possession became theirs.

Individual ownership is a fact of American society, and there are laws against theft. Maybe fewer children will become shoplifters if ownership can be explained when they are young and if their early thefts are not ignored. I do not believe that they should be physically punished when they arrive home with candy bars from the store or pennies from the neighbor's table. Rather, we parents should accompany our children to return the stolen objects. This usually makes a powerful and not-to-be-forgotten impression on the child as well as the parent. Among our more vivid memories as parents are those occasions when we have had to accompany each of our children on that awesome walk to the feet of a store manager.

Nursery Schools

Each of our children had nursery school experiences, and we felt it was good for them as well as for their parents. At this entry, Anne was almost four and Joy was three-and-a-half.

April 28—I am now letting Anne and Joy make their own sandwiches in the morning because they have complained about any variety I make even if it was made at their request. They prefer their own creations.

I visited Joy's nursery school class this morning. All seemed in chaos except Joy, who sat calmly occupied in placing national flags on maps of Europe and Asia. She didn't notice me until fifteen minutes had passed by. How she beamed, ran to me, showed me some cards with pictures of presidents and held my purse out to me when I said that I had to leave. She struck me as the most well-adjusted child there. How amazing! We returned home, and I complimented her on her behavior in nursery school. The children ran to take naps immediately, for they had been promised a trip to visit Daddy at his office.

Children can have good times in nursery school. They can learn to socialize with their peers and with adults other than parents. They can practice a few skills such as dancing, singing, and climbing, which they enjoy at a certain level of motor development. They can have available paints, brushes, hammers, nails, sand, etc., which they can use creatively when they feel like it. They can learn about consideration for the wishes of others and about sharing.

A good nursery school experience is a tremendous advantage to most children. It can be of particular benefit to children from homes that are disadvantaged in one way or another. However, children of upper socio-economic levels are more likely to have the nursery school experience. The nursery school concept has been accepted earlier in many European countries and in formerly colonial African and Asian countries than it has in the United States.

Nursery schools in the United States are accredited on the basis of cleanliness, space and safety. Since there is no uniform base on which to determine quality, parents tend to choose on the basis of where neighbor children go, the recommendations of other parents, books which espouse certain methods, convenience of location and time schedules.

Some nursery schools emphasize creativity more than structure. Others, such as Montessori, tend toward a more structured approach. Our experience is that the theory matters not nearly so much as the personality and warmth of the teachers. Qualities of love for children, kindness and flexibility can make almost any theory a good one in practice. Some nursery schools are operated as business ventures and could not exist if they did not return a profit to their investors. Ironically, suburban nursery schools tend to be both affordable and profitable because many highly skilled women are willing to teach in them at very low salaries. It is also unfortunate that male teachers are still so rare in nursery schools. If salaries were higher, children might have the benefit of a more balanced perception of the sexes in their nursery school experience. But if the cost of nursery schools were to go up, it would be harder to afford.

Parents should be aware that children are likely to catch many upper respiratory infections during their first year of school whether it be nursery or grade school.

One final note: We gradually learned that it was best not to plague the child for details of the day's activities at nursery school. The child should be allowed to "have his own thing" and to do any recounting on a voluntary basis.

Siblings

Siblings who are close in age usually find abundant reasons to squabble. They also defend, help, laugh with and love one another.

Siblings

Some of us grow up to consider our brothers and sisters to be our dearest, closest friends. I wish this for our four. At present, however, their relationships are far from mature:

> June 15—Anne and Joy got into a squabble over a doll after breakfast, and Daddy banished both to the playroom. Shortly after they entered the playroom, Anne got Joy to quiet down by giving her dozens of toys. Anne doesn't like to hear Joy crying and resents parental attempts to ignore the crying or tantrums. She is quite adept at calming Joy, but unfortunately the effect usually comes through placation. This could create problems in their sibling relationship as both get older.

It is regarded as a positive sign when children try to prevent parents from disciplining their siblings, or intervene when neighbor children mistreat siblings. This indicates that they are developing love and concern for one another, and this must antedate love and concern for others in the community. Sometimes siblings may become more protective than parents, and a younger child may be denied independence by an ever-present, watchful elder sibling.

Bedmaking is supposedly part of the morning rituals for our children. I have spent time with each one carefully demonstrating bedmaking. Months went by before I knew that Joy rarely made her own bed. Anne quietly made both. Now that Anne does not find bedmaking such a delight, she is annoyed when Joy asks her to make her bed.

Which child is better prepared for adulthood? The younger sibling whose doting older sibling makes the bed? The only child whose doting parents never expect him to make his bed? The only girl who is expected to make her own bed and her brother's? Or should we just not bother about beds at all?

Much of the world's population have only a single mat to be concerned about. If making or not making a bed will affect a child's perceptions concerning his dependence, the role of the sexes, and relative importance—it might be better to forget about it.

And if an ever-present, watchful, doting elder sibling seems to be preventing independence in the younger child, it might be wise to arrange for separate activities for the elder.

Win or Lose

Everyone likes games. In primitive cultures people devise games using the sticks and stones they find lying around. In the Western world we like to spend a fortune buying our games in pretty boxes.

I have enjoyed all kinds of games—verbal games, ball games, card games, chess—but most of all, the games I've played with my children.

> July 18—As the children and I drove to the hospital this morning, we played the "symphony game." I turn on the classical music station and begin, "Can you guess the story in this music?" The children take off with wonderful descriptions of dancing bears or flying ducks, and I chime in whenever I can. Beethoven may never have dreamed of the stories he would trigger in the heads of children.

This game has no win or lose aspect, so it is not threatening to young children. I fear that we introduced our kids to win-lose games before they were ready for them.

> July 18—When all three of the children are together, there are frequent episodes of quarreling. Now we have

six swings outside, and they manage to quarrel over who will use a particular one. Seems impossible. After supper tonight, I played checkers with Peter while the girls kibitzed; and later we all played Old Maid. Peter cried when he lost at checkers.

"If I am special and can do special things, why don't I win all the time?"

There are win or lose aspects to most games, active or sedentary, which children begin playing at three or four. Children may not recognize the winner-loser concept consciously when they play tag, hide-and-seek, blindman's bluff; but they do recognize it when they learn card games, chess or checkers. This can be a very difficult time.

What do we do when a child throws the checkers on the floor because he has lost? If our own composure is intact we explain that everyone loses sometimes, but that we learn by losing, and that we might win next time. And the game is put away until the child has regained composure.

My own observation is that the ability to lose with grace does not appear much before seven or eight and, of course, may never arrive at all.

Morning Madness

Those of us who work full-time sometimes complain about the pressures or the necessity of working nights and weekends. I am no exception; but unlike some of my male colleagues, I remember exactly how it was when I was at home full-time with toddlers, or how it was when I was working part-time at the office and full-time at home.

October 19—Yesterday morning I worked at the office

and did not arrive home until about ten minutes after Peter's kindergarten bus arrived.

"Were you feeling lonesome?" I asked.
"Naw," said Peter. "I had a peaceful, quiet time." (His father's phrasing.) "I liked it."

I also worked this morning, and there was the usual rush-rush to get all of us out. Daddy leaves at 7 a.m. When he leaves I ask the kids to get dressed—serve them breakfast—ask the kids again to finish dressing —put Joy in the tub—soak her sheets in soapy water —get myself ready for work—remind Joy to eat—tell Peter to feed the dog—ask Anne to put her shoes on—tell Peter to let me tie his shoes—dress Joy—ask them to put coats on—put dishes in the dishwasher—put things in the refrigerator—turn off the lights and, with luck, drive out by 8:20. I feel as if I've done a day's work by the time I arrive at my peaceful office to relax with only one child at a time.

The activities of the house-person vary considerably depending on the number and ages of children. But having a number of pre-schoolers, even though they may be in nursery school several mornings a week, keeps one hopping. My husband and many other men who, like him, have tried housekeeping and child care agree.

Money Sense

References to money have begun to show up in the diary. Peter is going on six and Anne is past her fourth birthday.

August 22—I picked a pail of apples a few days ago and

put a dozen or so in a paper bag and told the kids that they could take them to a little neighbor girl who has broken her arm. I was on the phone when they left. The next morning I discovered my empty pail and realized that they had taken all the apples to the neighbor. Now I understand why the neighbor had called to thank me profusely for "all those apples."

Peter was very helpful yesterday. He unloaded the dishwasher, fed the dog, vacuumed the rug and the sofa cushions. Anne helped to bake pies and Joy made her own bed. The children went with Daddy to deliver the garbage and to get groceries. Daddy told me that Peter spent all of his two-week accumulation of allowance on a birthday present for me. Money is suddenly becoming meaningful to the children. Anne asks me for pennies and has her own little hoard. Peter asks to open a bank account.

October 24—Anne is now aware of the value of money. When I took the girls shopping on Thursday morning she had an accumulation of twenty-seven pennies, which a friend had given her. She asked to buy a card of buttons (pink, of course), and we did that. We worked on sewing one doll dress this afternoon, and then she lost interest in her buttons.

We tried the allowance system only briefly; when the children got a little older we switched to a system of paying wages for family chores performed. A chart on the refrigerator door was cluttered with the accumulated debits and credits for each child.

Even with an allowance system, it is a good idea to remind the child that the allowance comes in recognition that he is now a responsible member of the family who will share responsibility for simple family tasks. With the allowance system, however, it is probably not a good idea to withhold the money on the basis of bad behavior or failure to do a family chore.

We have tried to give the children the option of deciding what to do with their own money. But we do throw in an occasional veto. We encourage saving, and once in a while we get talked into giving an advance on future earnings. The latter can lead as easily to misunderstanding with children as it can in the adult world.

If family fortunes decline, so can the allowance—especially if the facts are explained. While it is unwise to load a child with the full weight of our adult financial burdens, most children would be very proud to be included in a general family belt-tightening. I remember this sort of experience from my childhood and feel it was a maturing one for my siblings and me.

Going to the Dentist

Some adults suffer an emotional trauma that began in a dentist's chair in childhood; and to them, going to the dentist always seems a dreaded event. This need not happen. If we can keep from projecting our own fears on the children, they can get off to an early positive start. Anne and Joy were four and three when they made their first visit.

> August 22—Yesterday was another long day of errands. The kids and I left home at 8:45 a.m. First to Children's Hospital, where I signed some charts; then to see the ophthalmologist, who gave a good report on Peter's eyes and said that he would not need to see Peter again for six months. After that we went to the zoo for about two hours in the ninety-degree heat. We

> spent much time looking at the bears and snakes, then sat on the grass and ate our lunch. We went on to take Anne and Joy to visit the dentist for the first time. Anne had one cavity, which was discovered on the x-ray, and Joy had three. That bothered me because Peter has had no cavities so far. The girls were charmed by the pedodontist, as Peter had been. We arrived home around four, too late for naps, made supper, and the children went to bed early.

Children will often respond positively to a simple suggestion by their parents that new and different feelings in the mouth from dental work need not bother them. If they do not expect to gag or to find suction or x-rays uncomfortable, they may find these experiences quite comfortable. Calm, thoughtful parents can help prepare the child for a good experience, which should occur if the dentist is skilled with children.

In a sense, parents prepare children for the dentist by the diet they feed them, by whether or not they teach tooth brushing, leave bottles in bed with toddlers at night, and whether or not they use fluoridated water or fluoride pills. A diet low in sweets together with regular tooth brushing and fluoride will decrease cavities and, therefore, the need for any potentially painful procedures in the dentist's office. The initial visit will be easier if parents choose a pedodontist—a dentist who specilizes in children—or a general dentist who particularly enjoys working with children.

Ethical Sense

Most parents will agree that a little conscience is good and desirable. Its beginnings are apparent very early. Guilty faces are noted on two-year-olds who have picked up a "no-no."

Ethical Sense

Four-year-olds try to cover up their misdeeds in clumsy fashion, but they may continue to repeat the same acts. Conscience has arrived when a five- or six-year-old restrains himself from carrying out an unkind impulse or suffers guilt feelings when he does find himself yielding to it. Six- and seven-year-olds follow rules when they play with their peers or find themselves excluded from the games. They not only have their own conscience, but they may become the conscience of their parents. "Daddy, you're going past the speed limit." "Mama, you forgot to say please."

Peter was close to six when the following incident occurred:

> September 14— During the past weekend Peter acted as though something was bothering him. He was obviously unhappy, irritable, and his personality seemed so changed that I actually wondered if he could be developing a brain tumor. Yesterday morning I found out why. He said, "I don't want to go to school."
>
> "Why?"
>
> "Well, I didn't like school, so I messed up the dollhouse —(pause)—but I put it all back together. I was mad and messed it up."
>
> I asked, "Was it you alone?"
>
> "No, some other boys and I did it."
>
> He added that one of the older neighbor boys had told him on Saturday that he would be getting some kind of demerit or punishment from the teacher.
>
> I said, "Peter, if the teacher has any problem with you she'll call me." There was a long silence. He said, "Do they have your phone number?" "Yes, the school has all our phone numbers, including my work number and Daddy's work number."
>
> "Did they call you?" he asked nervously.

"No," I said. "Peter, I think the reason you've been so unhappy all weekend is that your conscience has been bothering you for messing up the dollhouse. So I'll tell you what to do. You go to school and tell Mrs. White that you're very sorry and will not do it again. Everything will be all right."

So he went to school and came home happy as a lark. He said that he had apologized, and Mrs. White had told him that he could use the dollhouse again. I received a nice note from Mrs. White which said that Peter was the only child involved in the dollhouse incident who had apologized and that she appreciated our help.

Along with conscience comes more maturity and independence. Children may resent and resist admonitions and instruction from parents as they develop their own guidance systems. But acquiring an ethical sense is worth a considerable amount of growing pains.

The expectation of parents, teachers and counselors that their children will have good value systems and ethics is important. Statements like "You're a liar" or "You're a thief" can too easily become a self-fulfilling prophecy.

Imaginations

The imaginations of children are marvelous resources, not only for themselves, but also for their parents. Here are Joy, Anne and Peter at three, four, and almost six.

September 22— I worked yesterday and the girls went happily to Mrs. Benke's, while Peter spent the day with Aunt Barbara. I picked the children up late in the afternoon and did some shopping for groceries on the way home. I felt really tired. Anne must have tuned in on my fatigue. As I drove in the driveway, she said, "Mama, you're tired. Don't get out. I'll do it." She got the mail, opened the gate, shut the gate, and then brought everything in from the car, including two heavy bags of groceries. I praised her immediately and again at suppertime, and I noted that Peter and Joy were outdoing themselves to be helpful after supper.

Last night, again, Peter mentioned several times that one girl in his kindergarten class has moved into first grade. In fact he said to me, "I think on Monday I'll do everything my teacher says, and then she'll put me into first grade." I asked if he had been acting badly. He said, "On Friday I played with Tinker Toys when she didn't want me to." Poor Peter.

He seemed a little sad at bedtime, and I talked about it while he was going to bed. "Peter, sometimes you're sad. Let's pretend it's a day when you're sad and you and I go for a walk." I described plants and birds and trees along the way. "Then we reach a beautiful garden." At this point Peter chimed in and described colors and plants and flowers. I said, "It's warm and cozy, and we feel so happy." By this time he had a big smile on and was asleep before I left his room.

I didn't have a ready answer for Peter's perception of a problem with respect to his desire to be in first grade instead of in kindergarten. In fact, when he mentioned it I didn't know if the girl who disappeared from his class had really gone to first grade, or moved away, or become ill. As a mother who had her eldest child in public school for the first time, I didn't know about policy with respect to skipping grades, etc.

I felt sad that my child was sad, and my approach on that particular evening was to divert his thoughts to a pleasant scene. It worked. It has worked for us many times when our children are sad and upset. I might add that I have not found myself able to divert the thoughts of a child so skillfully when the child is in the midst of a full-blown tantrum.

The imaginations of children are easily tapped. Their ease of visual imagery and their capacity to change their feeling state to match the imagery are wonderful qualities. Sometimes I ask my children to describe the pleasant scene, the lovely colors, the restful place; and their descriptions help carry me with them to calm, quiet and contentment.

Enuresis

Enuresis means urinating in an inappropriate place. Nocturnal enuresis is a euphemism for bed-wetting; and there is daytime enuresis and also a combination of both. These terms are not used for babies or toddlers who have not yet developed sufficient bladder maturity to have either daytime or nighttime control.

The age at which children develop bladder maturity varies tremendously. One of our children had daytime control at 15 months and nighttime control at two years. Another had daytime control at two and nighttime control at three. Another had daytime control at three and nighttime control at five-and-a-half.

> October 7—Joy arose at 6 a.m. and seemed to be in a cranky mood, so I persuaded her to return to bed until she felt more cheerful. She went back to sleep, got up in an hour in a pleasant mood, but absolutely soaking wet. She wears a terrific ammonia odor each morning

> and requires a bath before breakfast. In spite of plastic pants her sheets are also wet. I have put up a color chart for dry, half-dry, or no change; but she doesn't seem a bit interested. In fact she's taken it off the wall a couple of times.

When I made this diary entry I had two children who were already dry at night, and had been dry long before reaching Joy's age. I had not received any special training concerning the problem of bed-wetting during my pediatric training; and I, like many parents, expected that all the children would follow a similar pattern. Perhaps if Peter and Anne had continued wetting the bed until four or five, I would not have had such high expectations for Joy; thus I tried color charts and star charts. I know now that they were useless, because her bladder had not matured sufficiently to allow dry beds. I was tired of the morning baths, wet sheets, daily laundry; and my motivation was much greater than Joy's.

After some intensive study of the condition known as enuresis, I learned that twenty-five percent of children do not have dry beds until five or older. I wonder how much damage is done to children's self-image by parents or other relatives who expect them to be dry by age three or, perish the thought, even by two. A mother with children in the Washington D.C. school system told me that many children are beaten before they come to school by parents who are enraged over wet beds. Bedwetting has triggered child battering to the point of death.

When a child has reached the age of bladder maturation and has continuing nocturnal enuresis, he should be checked for urinary tract problems such as infection or abnormalities of anatomy. If these exist, they can be treated. If there are no infections or abnormalities, children can be taught to overcome the problem themselves.

Daytime dribbling or evidence that the child has a poor urinary stream, e.g., start and stop, is an indication for medical evaluation at any age, even infancy. The development of daytime or nighttime enuresis after the child has had a long period of bladder control is also an indication for medical evaluation at any age. The child who has had no dry beds—or only occasional dry beds—and never a sequence of dry beds lasting more than a week, can be expected to become totally dry by the time he or she is around six. If our expectations are reasonable, there may be no problem.

Although there are reports of punishment for and concern about enuresis in primitive cultures, it is likely that we Americans tend to regard it as more of a problem because it messes up our homes and because we have time to perceive it as a problem. It shouldn't be, anytime.

From the Mouths of Babes

The flashes of understanding that children show at a very young age are often among the most treasured memories we parents bring back from those consuming years of raising a family. Here's Joy at age three years and nine months.

> October 10—Yesterday all of us attended our church retreat, and the children had a good time. We planned to attend today, but Joy developed a croupy cough during the night, so I stayed home with her today while the others went back. She had intermittent fever today and slept three hours during the afternoon. When she was awake she sat in my lap and enjoyed concentrated maternal attention all day. She was literally clinging to me during all her waking minutes and did not at any time involve herself in personal play or activity apart

from me. She was quiet and pleasant until the others returned home. As I greeted them she screeched, "Mommy, Mommy, let me sit on your lap." Even though I knew she had sat on my lap for hours today, this plea always makes me feel that somehow I have withheld love from a child.

Shortly after they arrived she was sitting on Daddy's lap and he said, "Joy, would you rather get love or give love?"

"Rather get love," she said. "Giving love is too complicated."

Shortly after that, at 5:30 p.m., she removed her clothes and voluntarily went to lie in her bed. Later she ate a bit of supper, and is now lying on the sofa watching the fire.

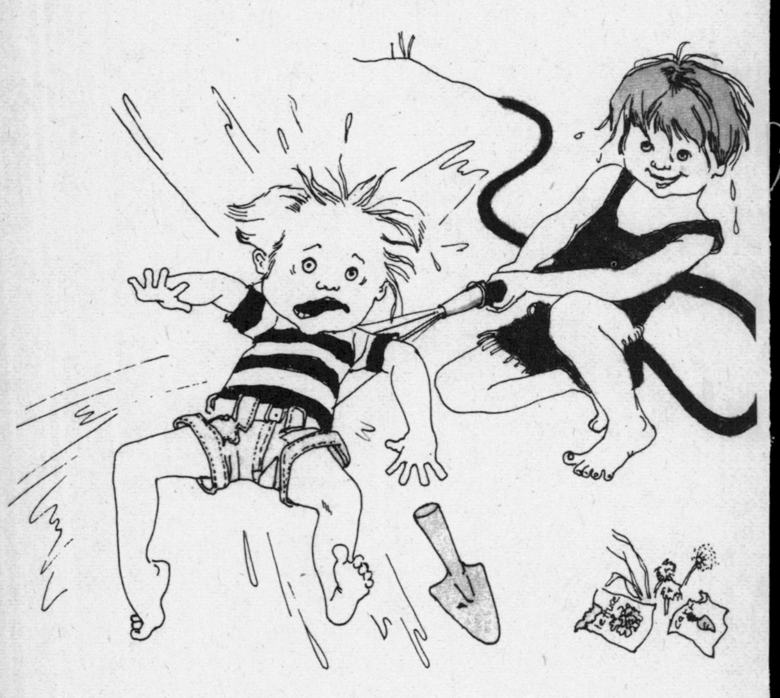

When involving children in work it is useful to remember that many do not have long attention spans.

5
Life with children aged four to seven

Peter was now six and in kindergarten. Anne and Joy were four-and-a-half and almost four and attending nursery school. I was still practicing medicine part-time; but by the end of the year my husband and I would have reached the decision to trade roles, he assuming primary responsibility for the children and the home, while I would pursue academic medicine full-time.

The Oedipus Complex

When I took college psych I not only heard about the Oedipus complex, I even saw the play, "Oedipus Rex." Intermittently throughout medical school, the Oedipus complex was discussed. I soon became bored with what I took to be a dubious theory—the theory that, at some point, boys wish to marry their mothers. Later, when Peter was six, I learned that the theory had some substance.

> January 8—Tonight I was in Peter's room, sitting on the guest bed and supervising his undressing.
> "Put your belt away. Now put your clothes in the linen hamper," etc.
>
> When his pajamas were on he said hesitantly, "Mama,

I don't know how to say this. It sounds funny." At this point he ran to me, threw his arms around me and said, "But I love you and I want to marry you."

I said I was pleased, that I loved him, and that I wouldn't be upset when he comes to me some years from now and tells me he is marrying someone else."
"No, I'll never do that," said Peter.

I was better prepared three years later. Here at ages nine and six are Peter and his brother Keith, who had joined our family by then:

February 16—Sunday morning and, as usual, I stayed in bed a little longer—until at least 8 a.m. Peter was already hard at work on his pancake making when I awakened. After awhile Daddy hopped out of bed to make tea; and almost immediately, Keith, standing in the doorway, hopped in.
Daddy said, "I can't stand this Oedipus complex. It's too much for me."

Peter, arriving at the bedroom door with a tray of pancakes, said, "What's the Oedipus complex?"
I said, "There's an ancient story about a son who wanted to marry his mother, and his name was Oedipus. And it's thought that boys sometimes want to marry their mothers, and we call it the 'Oedipus complex.' You said you wanted to marry me when you were around six or seven."
Peter absolutely denied it. "I didn't, and I don't want to marry you now."

I could hardly keep a straight face when Keith said seriously, "But now I want to marry you, Mama. And I will."

Keith has already changed his mind; and each of our children by age seven or seven-and-a-half was wrapped up in a school love affair, talking of marrying this girl or that boy. That stage also lasted for only a few months.

It helps to have had experience with previous children when these stages come along. I suspect that many of us laugh at such statements from our children, and that such a response is disappointing and deflating to them. On the other hand, it's probably not a good idea to give evidence that we take them seriously and, in doing so, reinforce their decision to marry Mommy or to marry Daddy or to marry the seven-year-old girl next door.

Heal Thyself

Pediatricians' families can be unglued by illness as much as any other family, especially when the pediatrician in the family gets sick, too.

> January 15—Everyone is asleep and sick. For the first time that I can recall, everyone in the family is sick at the same time. Even I am at least touched by a flu syndrome. Anne awakened Thursday saying that she couldn't walk because her legs hurt. She had a fever all that day and wouldn't eat at all. Joy became ill at school on Friday, and I picked her up from school at 10 a.m. She lay on the sofa all day, very feverish and refusing all food and drink—even Coke. It hit Daddy around 4 p.m. Friday, and he's complaining of a sore throat, cough and aching. Peter developed a cough during the night and I had chills. Today I feel congested, tired, and the chills continue. Peter seems the sickest and remained in bed all day.

Anne, feeling better, was very helpful today; even prepared breakfast in bed for Daddy (a carefully buttered toast and peanut butter). Peter asked me for some attention tonight. He said, "When Joy was sick you said that the sick person gets the most attention. Now remember that, and give me some." It's tough to keep that commitment when we're all sick.

Television and Movies and Small Children

Pre-school children in the United States sit for the schooling provided by television and movies for what is now estimated to be an average of 54 hours per week. Many parents, pediatricians, nursery school teachers and psychologists are worried about the negative effects from this "school." But most of us have television sets in our homes, and we yield to the requests of children to let them watch the tube and to take them to movies. I grew up without TV. I saw my first movie when I was nine years old. Yet I have allowed my children to watch movies earlier than I did, and to watch television.

January 30—Daddy flew to New York for one day yesterday. The children and I went to the movie, "Song of the South." The last time the children saw a movie was last summer with Daddy. The movie was "Pinocchio." Peter became so terrified that Daddy brought them home in the middle of the picture. This time Peter jumped into my lap three times when he identified too strongly with the boy in the movie, Johnny. Otherwise the kids did seem to enjoy it. Joy sat quietly, entranced throughout.

Television and Movies and Small Children

February 13—We got a new portable television last week, but somehow the kids haven't resumed watching "Sesame Street." The old set was on the blink for about two months before we replaced it, and the children seem to have lost the habit—just as well.

The information about the positive and negative effects of television is mostly speculative at this time, although a few good research studies have been completed. One such study indicated that ten-year-old children who watch violence on television do not react to real life violence as appropriately as children who do not watch violence. There are concerns that if children perceive that the person shot and killed on TV today appears again tomorrow, this might lead them to believe that bullets have no permanent effect.

If five-year-olds sit passively for 40 hours per week, do their large muscle groups develop less well? What about skills requiring eye-hand coordination? There is much evidence that the state which children reach while watching television is a very suggestible one. Note that my diary used the word "entranced" to describe Joy at the movies. Do our children realize consciously that they have been programmed by television commercials to harass us while we are shopping? What are the long-term effects of using television as a substitute for a bedtime story? Studies indicate that many children fall asleep either in the living room or in their own bedrooms while watching television. Are they more suggestible to whatever is on television as they pass through early sleep stages?

Until these questions are answered definitely, the most reasonable approach seems to be to watch what our children watch, decide if we as parents feel it is appropriate for them, discuss the programs with the older children, and make efforts to arrange family activities which are not so dependent on TV.

Our current solution (it might change by next week) is to

limit television to one hour a day and to give advance approval of the program chosen. If our children elect not to watch one hour a day, their money account is credited with twenty cents. Occasionally for a two-hour special they may use two days' worth of television viewing at once. This arrangement seems to be working, although not many twenty cents have been credited.

Mama is a Doctor

Despite our feeling that we were a well-liberated household, our children sometimes reflected culturally ingrained ideas about appropriate roles for boys and girls. In their games Peter tended to be the doctor and the pilot, while Anne was the nurse and the stewardess. And they could be intimidated by authority figures.

> February 13—Peter and Joy were sitting in my office today when Dr. Bob came by and, teasing, said, "Only doctors are allowed in here. This is a doctor's office." Immediately Peter and Joy looked stricken. Then Joy pulled herself together. Loudly she declared, "This is a doctor's office, and there is a doctor in here. My mama is a doctor." Everyone laughed. Peter looked relieved.

In contrast I recall the day when Peter was four and someone asked him what he wanted to be when he grew up. His classic reply: "I want to be a doctor. You know, boys can be doctors, too."

Studies of women who have become business leaders show that they had in common fathers who had high regard for them as whole persons capable of entering whatever profession they might choose. It never occurred to these girls before they started grade school that certain occupations were more appropriate for one sex than for another.

The expectations which parents have for their sons and daughters and which children have for themselves in early years seem to have a great influence on the course of adulthood.

It's Not Fair

With children aged four, going on five and six, it sometimes took more wisdom than I had at hand to keep petty sibling jealousies from marring otherwise beautiful moments with the kids.

> February 13—On our way home I picked up three boxes of valentine candy hearts (nickel boxes). Peter and Joy managed to eat their boxes plus Anne's before she came home from the birthday party. She was incensed when she found out and quickly asked me to buy her one-and-a-half boxes. Her logic: Peter had eaten his own and half of Anne's box and Joy had done the same. Therefore, in order to give Anne an equal amount, I should buy her one-and-a-half boxes of valentine hearts.

In spite of our parental platitudes—"Don't worry if someone else gets more," "Things can't always be equal," "Do you remember when you got something that Peter didn't?"—the children still watch intently when I cut a pie or a cake or bring home small gifts after a trip to ensure equality. My knowledge of this concern in young children has led me to remember the siblings in the waiting room when I offer a young patient a plastic ring or a tongue blade, etc. We must have done something wrong somewhere along the line to have made this a problem for our family. The mistake may have been to arrange for too many children too close together, all of whom have more or less similar interests and values.

To Change Behavior

Behavior modification systems were coming into vogue when a visit to the home of a psychiatrist friend started us toward a behavior modification program in our household.

> February 13—We noted the behavior charts on the refrigerator. They had been using this system for several weeks and found it very helpful for the children. So we decided to try. Our friends suggested we make a list of qualities which were important and valuable to us and to give our children pluses and minuses and stars for behavior that related to those categories. Our list included cooperation, kindness, smiling face, quiet voice, neatness, obedience, creativity, helpfulness, tooth brushing, hand washing, sharing. The charts have been in use for four days, and I do not notice any great improvement in behavior. In fact the only change is negative. The children detest getting minuses and threaten each other with minuses instead of "I'm going to tell on you."

We continued to use that system for about two months, and it gradually faded out of our consciousness. Actually, I think the April chart fell off the refrigerator door and no one noticed. Someone might well say, "Your children were too young for that. At four, four-and-a-half, and six, could they really comprehend what you were trying to do?" There are studies which show that very young children (age two and three) can respond to similar systems, but success requires much consistency and reinforcement. And it certainly requires motivation.

To Change Behavior

For our family it seems more effective to have a comfortable family sit-down together, to relax, and to have each of us imagine whatever the desired change in behavior is. The child decides what change is desirable; e.g., to finish schoolwork, to stop scraping chairs, to eat breakfast more quickly, to speak kindly to one's sister, etc. We all agree that it is possible, and we encourage our child or sibling to imagine the change and the good consequences from the change.

Acting Out or Reacting?

Peter at age six waited for the school bus at the bottom of the long driveway. One day we were appalled to hear from a neighbor that Peter had lain down in the middle of the road when he saw her approaching in the car.

> March 5—She told us she had "tongue-lashed" him, and said she would spank him if she saw him doing that again. This morning, almost first thing, Peter ran over Anne's toe with his bike because "she was in the road." Daddy took the opportunity to bring up our concern. Peter did not admit defeat immediately. With a cocky-sounding voice he said, "I like to do it." But shortly after Daddy left the kitchen, Peter came towards me with tears streaming down his face and proceeded to kick me. Daddy then put him in his room to think. I had said that we would wait for the bus every morning with him until he had matured enough to wait by himself.
> Tonight I chatted with him after he was in bed.
> "Peter, can you tell me? Will you lie down on the road again? If you feel that you will, we will stand by and wait with you for the bus. We will support you as long as you need it."

> "No, Mama." He said calmly. "I'm sure I won't."
>
> I went on to discuss how some of our mistakes affect only ourselves, but that the worst mistakes are those which affect not only us but people we love. Peter listened quietly; then said he understood.

Peter had complained about the teasing he had received from the older eight- and nine-year-old boys while he waited with them for the bus. Perhaps he was telling us that he wanted our support with him while he waited for the bus. But he soon assured us that he needed us no longer; and to the best of our knowledge, he has never repeated that particular performance.

Attention-getting device? Suicide attempt? Normal six-year-old behavior demonstrating the arrogance, boastfulness, invincibility that a six-year-old would like to feel? I wracked my brain to try to figure out exactly why he had chosen to react in such fashion. Our home life seemed happy, stable; and yet Peter was reacting to something.

Later I found out that the older boys had been lying down on the road demonstrating their bravery to the younger ones. Is that the real explanation? I remain uncertain. If I could explain the origins of half the actions of my children, I would be lucky.

Eating Habits

If you will backtrack in this book, you will find a section about the food habits of our children when they were younger; and it includes some rather dogmatic statements about eating and how to encourage young children to eat properly. Perhaps if my children had continued to eat all their meals at home, they would have continued to eat, and apparently like, whatever I served. Perhaps their natural maturational process would have led to difficulties anyway. When this entry was written in the diary, each of the children had had at least two years experience in nursery school or in kindergarten.

> April 30—Daddy and the children have gone to church. I stayed home, not so much because I craved privacy as because I have not had a day at home unbroken by travel for at least five weeks—and I just didn't want to get into the car this morning. I promised the children shrimp Newburg for lunch. Which brings me to the subject of their eating. For years I have prided myself on the fact that our kids eat everything well. There has been no need to coax or cajole or fix special items. They had eaten what was present—but all that has changed during the past six months. The phrases "Yuck" or "I don't like it" are heard daily. Anne and Joy use them more frequently. I have suggested that they not use those phrases lest they offend their hosts when they eat away from home.
>
> Anne has developed a particular dislike of onions. For a while we catered to this when we fixed Chinese food with onions. I made a separate pan with all the ingredients save onions. But recently she has refused her special dish and prefers "plain rice" with a little soy sauce. She also attempts to put salt or soy sauce on everything—just like Aunt Barbara and my dad. I try to discourage this.
>
> Joy's big problem meal has become breakfast. She resists all forms of cooked cereal—Ralston, Cream of Rice, oatmeal, Wheatena, whatever. Recently she has begun eating perhaps two or three tablespoons of

whatever hot cereal is present, and that is followed by yogurt or bread with a slice of cheese or meat. She has a penchant for bread. At times I hide bread to prevent her from taking slices all day long.

And Peter eats a tremendous amount of food, but he doesn't care for meat. This morning he ate four waffles. So did Daddy. By 10 a.m. he said he was hungry. None of the children will eat cabbage at all any more.

Last week Daddy fixed "Surkaal," a Norwegian cabbage dish. Daddy and I ate and ate and exclaimed over its merits. The children took not a bite. They do like hamburgers, spaghetti, plain rice, shrimp Newburg, peas, catsup, apples, chicken noodle soup, eggs, and any sort of desert. We seldom offer sweet snacks, but offer raisins, apples, oranges, bananas, nuts, carrot sticks, when they are hungry between meals.

After observing the limited kinds of food available in villages in Asia and Africa (limited particularly during certain seasons), I sometimes wonder if the behavior our children demonstrated above is because we offer too much variety. We also structure eating times. A study from the University of Iowa has indicated that children left to their own eating times will eat six times a day. In rural or tropical areas, children may have access to fruits, vegetables, nuts, etc., which makes snacking easy and routine. My diary entry indicates that I was troubled by my children's rejection of my food offerings. We have come to accept the fact that Anne doesn't like onions and Joy doesn't like oatmeal. We continue to dislike the idea of wasting food. Cabbage is currently in again for some of the children. And I keep telling myself that if the food available in the house provides good nutrition, the children will be well fed.

Work Responsibilities

There is evidence that we parents tend to raise our children the way we were raised, to discipline as we were disciplined, to set the kind of limits that were set for us. Probably when the confusion of multiple child-rearing theories overwhelms us, we draw from our subconscious childhood memories. And perhaps cultural differences exist, not so much from differences related to economics, climates, style of building, etc., but from nuances of child-rearing differences which have evolved over centuries.

This may seem to be a strange lead-in to the subject of young children and work responsibilities. In preparing this I contemplated my nieces and nephews, as well as my own children, and recognized immediately that each of the four families involved expects children to participate in tasks around the house. Personalities of the parents vary as do the personalities of the children, but all of the children do work in their homes. Here are our four-, five-, and six-year-olds:

> June 18—Peter spent much time this weekend involved in pretend play with Pooh Bear. He painstakingly made clothes for Pooh Bear. Strange, he didn't seem to care about doll play when he was two; at that time cars intrigued him. Anne has done much unsolicited work this weekend—picking up, mopping, vacuuming, etc. Peter helps very grudgingly lately, and Joy is very reluctant to do any tasks. Grandma sent money for potato bug picking, a penny a bug. Anne picked most of the 24 bugs which the kids found.

Obviously the enthusiasm for, or abhorrence of, doing jobs around the house varied with the age and stage of our children. The children enjoyed family working projects the most. Togetherness helps a lot. I enjoy baking sessions with our four children. We bake four desserts or breads at once. I move from bowl to bowl, helping to measure, giving an extra stir occasionally, and having fun with the children. Undoubtedly not every parent would think this is fun. It drives Daddy bananas.

Unfortunately the word "work" has become associated with drudgery. Work in its purest sense is activity which leads to the realization of an idea. If young children can perceive that work can lead to happy outcomes—e.g., apple pie—the work itself can be enjoyable. Young children imitate work. Three- and four-year-olds can spend hours a day doing housework in their pretend existence. A one-year-old works as he learns to walk—standing shakily, wobbling, two steps, falling, up again and, at last, the joyous outcome as he runs across a room.

How much or how little responsibility children feel for tasks around home depends on parental expectations. If parents believe, "I'll do it because it is so much quicker"—or "Let him play (failing to recognize that much of the play is work); he's only a child once"—the child may not react positively at six or twenty-six when offered responsibility.

How does one share work at home with children? Watch for signs of imitation of your activities and praise those imitations when children are two or three years old. When they become a little older, a little verbal logic helps. "Let's clean up the playroom (or make your bed) so we'll have more time to go swimming."

Positive reinforcement helps. Praise his bedmaking although the spread is not quite straight. When that clumsily arranged breakfast in bed is brought to you proudly for the first time, rave. The breakfasts and their arrangements get better.

After ages seven or eight, monetary reinforcement is often used. I am not much in favor of allowances predicated on certain jobs done or not done. But association between work and happy outcome is made more rapidly for a seven- or eight-year-old if she works to earn a specific object. That is desired.

When involving children in work it is useful to remember that many do not have long attention spans. If work is to remain pleasurable, parents should keep the working time reasonable. Fifteen minutes of scrubbing a table is enough for the average four-year-old. One hour of lawn-mowing is probably enough for an eight-year-old. If the whole family is involved in the same project, e.g., planting a garden, the length of time the children can be happily involved is probably longer. Even with all-day efforts there should be time for rest, diversionary play, snacks, etc.

Recognizing that children vary in their abilities, here are some suggestions for what children at various ages might do around their homes. W.S. means "with constant supervision." I.S. means "initial supervision until child has learned the task."

Age 4
Bedmaking W.S.
Scrubbing W.S.
Dusting W.S.
Pulling weeds W.S.
Vacuuming W.S.
Pick up room or playroom W.S.

Age 5
Baking W.S.
Feeding pets W.S.

Age 6
Washing car W.S.
Ironing W.S.
Setting table I.S.
Picking vegetables from garden I.S.
Taking out garbage I.S.
Scrubbing I.S.
Bedmaking I.S.
Dusting I.S.

Age 7
Cooking W.S.
Carpentry W.S.
Cleaning barn W.S.
Feeding larger animals I.S.
Planting garden I.S.
Doing dishes I.S.

Age 8
Laundry I.S.
Lawn mowing I.S.
Raking leaves I.S.
Watering the garden I.S.

While reviewing this chapter early one Saturday morning, I was called to breakfast by my eight-year-old daughter. As I sat down to eat I noted that she was already busily doing the dishes (everyone else had finished breakfast), and our ten-year-old son was vacuuming the living-room rug. Joy had made her bed beautifully and was searching the house for returnable bottles. Keith was busy making his bed. They were obviously happy and content, chattering about their plans for the day, which included a birthday party for the girls and fishing for the boys.

Of course there are times when we hear, "I wish we had a maid" or "Why do beds have to be made?" or "I think I'll sleep in my sleeping bag all the time" or "Joy didn't do her share of the dishes." We have tried different techniques with respect to some of the recurring household tasks. Children have taken turns doing breakfast dishes or supper dishes. Currently our rule is: "Put your own dishes in the dishwasher and scrub two pots and pans or serving dishes." Daddy or I do what's left, and sometimes that is most of the dishes.

On the positive side, Peter can cook very satisfactorily and also safely drives the lawn tractor to do the lawn. Some readers might raise eyebrows at that. Once again my own upbringing on a farm is reflected in my expectation that he can be depended upon to drive the lawn tractor safely. Anne can do all aspects of housework very well. As we say, no one can mess up more or clean better than Anne. Joy can bake bread with minimal supervision. We share the usual recurring tasks of running a house, and we share the joys of recreation together. It works for us more often than it doesn't, so we recommend it. Other families may have better ways for their particular needs.

Rates of Development

Dr. Jerome Kagan, professor of Human Development at Harvard University, has written, "During the first few years of life, when there are frequent maturational changes in basic competences, individual differences are just as likely to be the result of differences in rates of development as they are to be a product of experience."

Parents who believe that the environment for their several children is similar and that the experiences of their children are similar are often impressed with the differences in the children. Our two oldest seemed to acquire their competences and skills in a gradual fashion. We began to realize that Joy had a different system. She progressed from sitting to walking with scarcely a crawling movement between. She spoke so little at eighteen months that I took her for a hearing check, and suddenly she began speaking in complete sentences.

> July 2—Joy is four and continues to manifest the same sort of "no sign of any progress, followed by a giant leap forward" development. Last week she spontaneously began writing her whole name after, to our knowledge, never having written a single letter. She also began drawing human figures containing ten parts after having gotten no further than a mere circle before. She also indicates by spontaneous comments that she can read. If I sit down with Joy and a book, she insists that I must read to her. She obviously reads signs, and I sometimes come upon her reading aloud from a book. Swimming lessons began last week. She refused to put her head under water and just kind of stood in the water doing nothing. Today I noticed she was swimming.

Joy was our youngest for five years before we adopted our

fourth child. She enjoyed having things done for her, and this may help explain the sudden developmental leaps which did not seem to follow the usual trial and error we expect in children. Maybe she was practicing when I wasn't looking. Her pattern did seem to be repeated in many areas, and I tend to believe that she put things together in her head before she proceeded with the motor activity involved.

Family Games

There are some helpful books on play activities and diversionary activities for children; e.g., *What To Do When There's Nothing To Do.* As is probably true for many families, we noted that certain unique play activities evolved which were created by our children and us.

> July 16—Today, Sunday, hot again, Joy took two helpings of hot cereal, which is most unusual. I have bought packages of cold cereal this week for the first time in ages. Peter says, "I love you for buying that." And Joy refuses to eat it.
>
> We had guests today. As is now her custom whenever guests arrive, Joy whispers to me, "Mommy, will you put the boom-boom record on so I can dance?" Today I said we would wait until the guests had left. The children and I love to dance together, and each of us has a favorite dancing record. We have a wonderful time dancing solo or together. It's relaxing for me at the end of a day.
>
> Tonight we danced and we also played the "walking" game. I sit on the sofa and say, "Peter, walk clumsily like a one-year-old baby learning to walk."
>
> Or, "Anne, walk gracefully, like a pussycat."

Or, "Joy, walk joyfully as though you had just heard you were getting a barrel of gum."
Joy maintains that gum is her favorite thing.

I have enjoyed writing plays for the children and directing them. And, of course, the children have prepared their own drama productions. We have friends who do puppet shows together with a miniature stage constructed especially for their basement. A respected pediatrician tutor of mine once said, "Ask parents if they enjoy their children. Do they have fun with them? If they do they're probably on the right child-rearing track regardless of methods." I believe my tutor was right.

Parents' Night

Child rearing is physically and emotionally taxing, especially for the principal caretaker and especially when the children include several pre-schoolers or—as I hear from my peers who are parents of adolescents—several adolescents. We felt a need occasionally to spend an evening out, just the two of us, and left the children with babysitters. As the children have evolved into grade schoolers we have felt less need to "get away." But when we planned an anniversary celebration for the two of us at home, it didn't quite work out:

September 1—Last night we took the children and one of their cousins to the community swimming pool for a picnic. After the children returned home I showed them our album of wedding photos, and we had a "good night time." I kissed the girls and sang them each their favorite goodnight lullaby. Anne sang the lullaby back to me. I lay down with Peter for a few minutes and discussed his fear of being alone in his room and, reassured, he fell asleep immediately. Then Daddy and I prepared a special candlelight dinner celebration for ourselves. As we were finishing our main course, we remarked on how thoughtful the children had been in falling asleep so quickly. Just as we finished, two heads appeared in the dining room. "We smelled all that good food and we're so hungry." They were so cute that we set Anne and Joy up with ice cream at 9:30. They ate quickly and went off to bed.

Early Romances

It had been several years since I had read *The Child from Five to Ten* by Gesell and Ilg. When our oldest child reached seven I was surprised by his sudden interest in the opposite sex.

October 28—Peter announced on Thursday afternoon that he had a girlfriend and asked Grandma about arranging dates. He said, "I don't know much about this date business." He was determined to call his friend Mary, who had called him at home as soon as he arrived from school. I allowed him to call Mary although I was feeling a bit concerned over the intensity of his romance. Peter announced at the dinner table that he was in love with Mary.

Yesterday morning he talked about her again. I said, "Peter, it's good to have boyfriends and girlfriends, but you're too young to have dates and get married."

"I know that," said Peter. "Mary and I know we're not going to get married. We just want the kind of date where she visits me at my house and I visit her at her house if our mamas say it is okay."

He went on to explain that two other boys in his class had girlfriends, too, and that the kids in his class teased one of the boys who had actually kissed his girlfriend.

Peter called Mary again last night.

"Hello, is Mary there? This is Peter—her boyfriend."

Then, "Mary, when you come over we can play in my boys' club upstairs in the barn."

He asked me when she could come over. I agreed to Saturday and he was overjoyed.

November 5—Mary was here yesterday afternoon and played with Peter, Anne and Joy. Mary seemed demanding and bossy, and Peter acted subdued. I served snacks to the children later in the afternoon. After Mary's mother picked her up, Peter said he thought he was too young to have any more dates.

Since then we've been through very similar "seven-year-old crushes" three times. They seem to last for two or three weeks, during which time there is much talk of love and marriage and the phone is busy constantly. As quickly as they come, they go. And a year or so later the vehemence with which the child denies the story can be awesome. So we parents have a taste of things to come.

I Hate You—I Love You

We recall how genuinely hurt poor Daddy felt the first time our eldest said, "I hate you. You're mean." Just as we have become accustomed to the seven-year-old loves, we have become accustomed to the six- and seven-year-olds' ambivalence about us and other authority figures. Here are Anne and Peter at five and almost seven:

> November 26—Anne was alternating hating and loving me tonight at bedtime.
>
> "Mama, I hate you." That was when she felt that I wasn't singing loudly enough.
> Later, "Mama, I love you."
> At one point this weekend Peter said, "I hate you, Mama."
> And, a few minutes later, I found a hand-lettered sign on my bedroom door, "I love you, Mama. Love, Peter."

I am perplexed over the source of the phrase, "I hate you." It appeared in our family after nursery school experiences, and its use seemed to peak around six or seven. Regardless of whether or not the children knew the word, the feelings of anger and frustration and guilt would appear at times, and the manifestation might be crying or hitting or the phrase, "I hate you."

Sometimes I would try to express their feelings for them. "You feel upset, you feel angry—it's okay to tell us that. I don't think you really hate us."

Eventually we learned to ignore it just as we learned to ignore the tantrums, the threats to run away, and the missing socks.

Inborn Traits

The fifth diary year had ended. A few weeks into the new year, when Peter was seven, Anne was five-and-a-half, and Joy was five, I wrote:

January 14 and 27—The diary doesn't get kept as often any more. I am busier, and the kids are changing less frequently. Anne has been begging to take ballet. Joy says she doesn't want ballet, although her spontaneous dancing shows that she is copying the ballet she has seen. Joy now has few tantrums, and she hasn't wet the bed for two months. Peter comes into bed with us each morning, but very briefly, because he is compulsive about getting ready for school on time. He likes to get down to the bus stop twenty minutes ahead of time . . .

Anne developed a runny nose on Tuesday night, then a fever and sore throat on Wednesday night. Throat culture was positive, and now she is on penicillin. She enjoyed the extra attention, but never really slowed down even when her fever was high. She is sturdy and invulnerable. Joy has been sleeping in Peter's room since Anne got sick. Tonight Peter lent her his pajamas, and I laughed to see the familiar pajamas on her more rotund configuration.

It sounds like things are all going smoothly—but not always so. Our discipline problems revolve around the necessity of eating all one has taken to eat at breakfast. The other major problem involves turning off the television when supper is ready. Peter is the chief offender and has had episodes of stamping and crying over this. Daddy gets most aggravated at the kids when they refuse food, saying, "I don't want it" or "I don't like it," and when they tell tales on one another. I get most aggravated by messiness and carelessness with clothes. When I ask Peter where his new gloves are and he replies, "I don't know. Maybe I left them at school"—that response triggers anger in me. I guess it must be clear to the kids that the mittens can be replaced in spite of my insistence that Peter earn his own money to replace them.

Looking back on the years described in the diary, it is easy to see the children developing through their experiences and through the expectations that their parents and others had of them. I am also struck by the development of the innate and unique personality traits of each child which continued to assert themselves without much evident regard for the child's experience of our expectations. The diary refers to Peter's obsessive-compulsive nature about time (definitely not about neatness or finishing projects), to Joy's spontaneous copying of ballet postures (she seems a born mimic), and to Anne's resiliency.

The personalities of our children may be very different from those of their parents, and these personalities may complement each other or clash. Or the personalities of a parent and a child may be very similar, and this similarity can be a problem or a blessing.

Obviously, children with innate differences will react differently to the same environmental influences. An innately trusting child is more likely to make a positive assumption about his or her environment than an innately more suspicious one. On the other hand, the latter child, having come to some assumption about the world, might endure more assaults on that assumption without abandoning it.

Take for example the personalities of children at age two—an age that has traditionally been described as hyperactive, negative and demanding. But these qualities vary greatly among two-year-olds, depending on the innate personalities and intelligence involved.

Each of our children showed increased activity and exploration around age two. This was most pronounced with Peter and least so with Joy. Peter was active in utero, and he was not a cuddly baby because he was constantly straining to lift himself up, to stand (even at six weeks) and to see his world. His attention span has always seemed shorter than that of the girls. At two, Joy might sit with a picture book for thirty minutes, while Peter would toss it aside for new frontiers after five minutes. Anne was a very cuddly baby who seemed to melt into my arms, and she would gladly cease her two-year-old's explorations to sit and cuddle for long periods.

Each of the children had temper tantrums. Peter's were loud but short-lived, and his "terrible twos" lasted only a few months. Anne had such mild tantrums that they could scarcely be recognized as such. Joy, on the other hand, was a master of temper tantrums. She was, when we first knew her at six months, suspicious of new situations and slow to adapt to them. She is strong-willed, and her negativism at age two could be fierce and unrelenting. We have postulated that these qualities kept her alive in the orphanage where many of her peers under twelve months of age died.

Some child development researchers have suggested that there is a category of "the invulnerable child." These are the rare children who have survived what most of us would think of as intolerable deprivation or an unbearable series of physical and emotional calamities. In spite of it all they manage to grow up into happy, coping adults. At the other end of the scale there are other exceptions—those who seem to fail despite having been nurtured in what we believe to be an excellent physical, emotional and spiritual environment.

The reasons for these exceptions are probably as numerous as the exceptions themselves. The innate characteristics of the child are no doubt an important factor. But when we look for a common factor, the one that seems to fit best is the factor of expectation. When I have seen a patient who seemed to fall into the category of the "invulnerable child," I have often discovered that the child or someone close to the child has an unshakable commitment to an expectation of life which denied the visible reality.

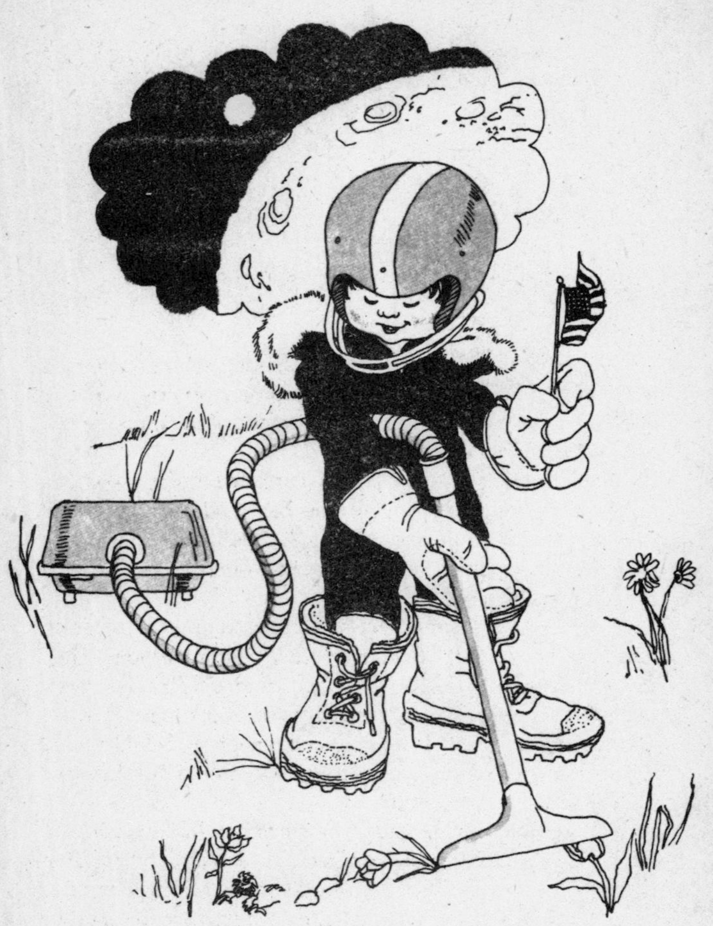

Toward the end of these diary years, we have come to realize that outcomes tend to conform to our unspoken expectations of one another and that our positive expectations are more important than our specific methods.

Positive Expectations

We all begin with our innate traits, but that's not where all the action is. The change, the development and the magic of growing up occur within the environment of our experiences and our thoughts.

A child who comes to feel at an early age that the world is, on balance, a friendly, loving one has made a giant stride toward growing into a happy adult. A child who comes to feel that the world is, on balance, against him has heavy odds against growing up happy.

The factors that influence the early assumptions that form in a child's mind are hard for an adult mind to fathom. They may not even seem logical to an adult mind. Children are more open to suggestions from themselves or from others than are adults. The thoughts and experiences that fill a child's mind have a far more powerful impact than do similar thoughts and experiences of most adults.

Those of us who are adults like to think that we came to adulthood through a process of learning and expanding. That was only part of the process. We were also contracting and forgetting. As we matured we learned to narrow our creative imaginations and to reject some of the suggestions that come from our own minds and from others.

In the television series "The Ascent of Man," Dr. Jacob Bronowski spoke with awe of the accomplishments of the great civilizations of the world. But he continued with this statement:

"And yet by one test they all fail — they limit the freedom of the imagination of the young."

If there is a "magic box" to aid in solving problems of child rearing, it is not a method at all, but an attitude ... an attitude in both the children and in their parents that frees the imagination to create expectations of the desired outcomes.

Again a thought from Dr. Bronowski: "... but magic is only a word, not an answer ... It says that man believed he had power, but what power? ... I think that the power that we see expressed here for the first time is the power of anticipation, the forward-looking imagination."

Children do this naturally. For adults it often requires abandoning well-established patterns of negative thoughts or expectations.

Consider this story of a patient, a boy almost four years old — beautiful, intelligent, asking and imagining, but picking up confused signals. His mother is very intelligent, married multiple times, a thief and an alcoholic. His father was a drug addict. His foster mother perceived him as brain damaged because of his hyperactivity and frequent destructive outbursts.

All three said they loved him. Professional consultants intellectualized correctly that he was reacting to changes in homes and caretakers and the instability of those caretakers. But neither their professed love nor cognitive understanding of his problem could help the boy. Could the natural mother conceive of herself in a stable enough situation to provide a happy, stable home for the boy? Could she imagine him a gifted, competent adult? Could the foster mother, or I the physician, or you the reader see the natural mother rebuilding a stable life and home? Could the foster mother see herself providing an interim of love and comfort for the boy? And could the boy see himself as intelligent, stable, and having the power of a forward-looking imagination?

Does the mother have any imagination left? And the foster mother? And the rest of us? And the boy ... surely his is still there if the limits set on it by fear, anger and anxiety can be lifted. The temptation is to say that it is too late for these imaginations. In saying that, we prove only that our own imaginations are weak.

Consider another boy, a patient aged seven, who is highly intelligent, performing in superior fashion at school and talking about his plans to become a physician. He also is from a broken home. His father abandoned him when he was two, and his mother has had several children by various fathers since then. Her presence in their changing series of apartments is sporadic. The boy has learned to cook, but there is not always food to cook. In addition, he is sometimes ill with eczema and asthma. He comes into the office clean, face shining, and his grandmother glowing beside him. "I have faith in this boy," she says each time she brings him for a checkup. "He will make something of himself." As the years pass we see him blossom. He fulfills her expectations.

I have come to believe that our expectations, be they positive or negative, translate themselves into realities. This seems to occur with all the precision we associate with the term "formula." The difficulty is that when I state my belief as a formula it comes out something like, "If you make certain that each of your thoughts about your child is positive, then child-rearing will be a breeze." But this is as unhelpful as all the other child-rearing prescriptions, or more so. So instead of a prescription or formula, I will offer a few additional examples and suggest that the reader consider them, adapt them, and perhaps develop his or her own way of increasing positive outcomes.

Example one: Most of us parents believe that we should

not leave children unattended at home. But suppose some situation arises in which a parent feels compelled to leave them briefly; e.g., your female dog in heat has escaped and you must try to catch her, or a neighbor needs help in an emergency. Now, what do you do? If you consume yourself in worry during the necessary errand and imagine all the possible disasters which might occur in your absence for which you would be responsible, the kids might tune in on that and make the disaster happen.

On the other hand, if you are relaxed, calm and have faith in your offspring to cope with the situation and perhaps to act a little more maturely in this unexpected absence, they are likely to do so. How do you relax, remain calm and think positively? Do it deliberately! Close your eyes for a few seconds if necessary in order to be able to imagine your coping children doing just that. Imagine something that's real for you — that they are eating breakfast peacefully and that you can see them dressed appropriately. Feel as you do when you are pleased and happy about an outcome, and confidently communicate this expectation. A parent can practice doing this and then it will seem much easier than imagining them playing with matches or getting into a fight.

Example two: If our own parents and grandparents have had many physical illnesses and have made us aware of them, we tend to expect these in ourselves and in our children. Thus, a routine cold can be seen as a base from which pneumonia might develop (Grandma had pneumonia many times and it always started with a cold), or an occasional loose stool might suggest that ulcerative colitis is on its way, or a tummy ache might mean ulcers or cancer. Not only might our child recognize that symptoms are more worthy of solicitous attention than is the healthy state, but the child might tune in on our anxiety and develop the anticipated illness. At other times the child remains fine and the parent becomes ill. I recall an instance when a parent (allergic himself) was consumed by the worry that his child would have a violent allergic reaction to a necessary penicillin injection. During the ride home from the doctor's office the parent broke out in generalized hives. Fortunately, he was able to recognize what had happened. It is worth considering and contemplating the possibility that some symptoms and illnesses are the result of self-fulfilling prophecies (expectations).

What might you do to avoid this? When your child becomes ill, imagine him as the special, sturdy person whom you know so well to be engaged in an activity which he enjoys when he is well. Do not ignore the illness or symptoms — act appropriately with respect to the advice of your physician. But, when you have done those things, consider and expect a positive outcome rather than a negative one. When my child steps on a toothpick and gets a good half inch stuck in the bottom of his foot, I will get the toothpick out and begin soaks. Then I have the option of anticipating a horrible infection because that toothpick was dirty, or I can have the option of imagining him running about perfectly normally in a few days. I do not know how this works. If a parent has the expectation of some dreadful complication, does that parent subconsciously care for the foot in such a way that the infection is encouraged?

Are soaks forgotten? Do parents transmit anxiety to the child which somehow causes his immune system to work less effectively? Some day we will know the answers. For now, we can say only that positive expectations are realized as are negative ones.

With respect to those habits of our children which we feel are wrong or bad or damaging, it is very easy for many of us to continue thinking about those habits. We get upset about them, imagine them continuing, and feed our offspring's own negative feelings about himself and the habit. It is hard for me to bite my tongue with respect to such habits. From my practice I know how hard it is for many parents.

"Doctor, you're asking me to do the most difficult thing."

"I can't control myself — I just get so irritated at his nail-biting, or thumb-sucking, or bed-wetting."

Rational statements such as "No one ever died from thumb-sucking"—or, "Would it be important if your entire family were in the midst of an earthquake or some other disaster?"—don't help a bit. Changing parental expectations may help.

Example three: Perhaps your six-year-old son, or nine-year-old daughter, or twelve-year-old son still wets the bed. Can you relax and imagine him or her exclaiming joyfully over his dry bed? Over a week of dry beds? A month of dry beds? If you say that you cannot imagine even one dry bed, how about imagining that the child is grown and out of the house? It's barely possible that the bed-wetting will persist to adulthood, but it won't be your problem then, just as it never really could have been your problem. Expecting lack of success, counting the failures, saying "It's not working," (no matter what the method of therapy) is hindering your child. Imagining success, even if you must imagine it in the distant future, is helpful.

If you're still feeling uptight and can't get into easy positive imagining, consider following a method such as a relaxation exercise, a meditative exercise, or reading in a prayer book. When your inner self is calm, imagine the outcome you wish.

If you can't imagine specific outcomes then imagine general ones. Imagine it's a year from now. You're on vacation and thinking about how pleased you are with your child's behavior, development and interests. How pleased you are that he or she is happy and how nice it is to be his or her parent.

Why not give this a try? The coats on the floor, the lost library books or the tantrums have no great significance as isolated instances. But if they trigger negative expectations they may indeed be very significant. And, if you can't turn the crayoning on the newly papered wall into a positive thought — ask your mate or a close friend to help you. You'll be able to do it again tomorrow.

Example four: It helps to teach children to use their imaginations positively. Bedtimes can be made special by many little family rituals. One of these might be to sit quietly with your children and imagine hoped for, happy future events. Children can take turns describing a happy future event. Maybe it's the last day of school and successful completion of first grade. Maybe it's visiting grandparents who live some distance away. Maybe it's passing the beginning swimmer's course. Maybe it's learning to parallel ski or being able to read and enjoy it. And maybe it's all dry beds. Children learn to consider the possibility of successful outcomes and they also learn that those most important people, their parents, are focusing on successful outcomes for them, too.

Conclusion

Ideally the conclusion to this book is the conclusion that each reader draws from it. You are raising your children and we are raising ours. There are similarities and differences, and both are significant.

For me the conclusion is that in child rearing, as in many human undertakings, almost everything is relative. Our children are different. Each arrives with a unique set of innate characteristics, and each discovers the uniqueness of his or her life situation.

Parents are different. Rarely do two of us perceive the same problems in child rearing, and what one of us may see as a problem in one setting may be no problem at all in another setting. The last diary excerpts indicate that my husband and I each had our own particular favorites among the situations we chose to regard as problems. Yours may be much different and make as little sense to us as ours do to you.

Even medical science is relative. Since I began studying medicine nearly twenty years ago, many of the so-called "facts" of medicine have changed. I have tried to bring current medical "facts" into this book, but it is likely that some of these will also change.

While I recognize there are no absolute answers to questions about child rearing, much of this book does contain my specific advice, at least by implication. Few of us can refrain from trying to impose our views on others, and pediatricians are no exception. Since we are required to be decisive and correct in our 3 a.m. advice on croup or meningitis, this tends to carry over into a habit for decisive answers in child rearing, too.

But readers of this book will have found that when it came to the rearing of our own children we were far from decisive and consistent. I hope our lack of consistency will be more a source of comfort than a cause for dismay.

Conclusion

There is great appeal in simple answers to child-rearing questions. We found that we gained more from exploring the options in child rearing than from trying to apply specific techniques.

Toward the end of these diary years, we have come to realize that outcomes tend to conform to our unspoken expectations of one another and that our positive expectations are more important than our specific methods. Every family must develop faith in their ability to create their *own* parenting pattern in their own way, and to visualize their children maturing into happy, self-reliant and fulfilled adults.

The only specific advice I hope you will take has to do with expectations. Whether you are a parent or a teacher or a grandparent or an aunt or an uncle or a foster parent or a babysitter, here is my suggestion:

Stop for a few minutes in the business of your day. Sit down, close your eyes and visualize the child for whom you care. Visualize him as happy, coping, and showing all his strengths. Visualize him thus at as close a point in time as you can comfortably achieve in your imagination — today, tomorrow, next month or next year. Visualize him positively, and yourself the same way. Your expectations and your love can do more for your children than dozens of child-rearing books.

August 22, 1976